Tai Ji
Qi

Best Wishes Always

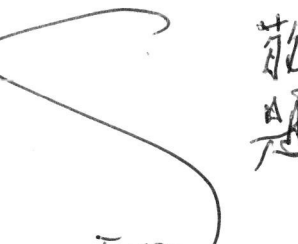

Chen Kung Series
From the Private Family Records of Master Yang Luchan

Tai Ji Qi

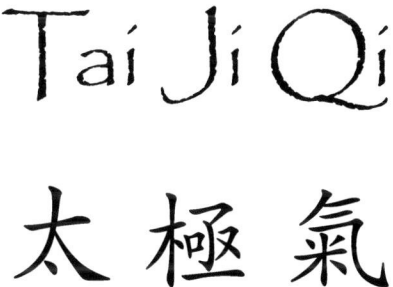

The Traditional Taijiquan Teachings on Qigong and Internal Alchemy

A New and Revised Edition of *Cultivating the Ch'i*

Translation and Commentary
by Stuart Alve Olson

Valley Spirit Arts
Phoenix, Arizona

Translations from *Tai Ji Quan, Sword, Saber, Staff, and Dispersing-Hands Combined* by Chen Kung (太極拳刀劍桿散手合編, 陳公著, Tai Ji Quan Dao Jian Gan San Shou He Lun, Chen Gong Zhe).

Disclaimer
Please note that the author and publisher of this book are NOT RESPONSIBLE in any manner whatsoever for any injury that may result from practicing the techniques and/or following the instructions given within. Since the physical activities described herein may be too strenuous in nature for some readers to engage in safely, it is advised that a physician be consulted before training.

Copyright © 2013 by Stuart Alve Olson.
Originally published by Bubbling-Well Press as *Cultivating the Ch'i* in 1986. Second Edition by Dragon Door Publications in 1993, and in 2005 as part of the book *T'ai Chi Qi & Jin* by Valley Spirit Arts. All rights reserved. No part of this publication may be reproduced or used in any form or by any means, electronic or mechanical, including photocopying, recording, or by any information storage and retrieval system, without prior written permission from Valley Spirit Arts.

Library of Congress Control Number: 2013932906
ISBN-13: 978-1-889633-15-2

Valley Spirit Arts
Phoenix, Arizona
www.valleyspiritarts.com
contact@valleyspiritarts.com

Dedication

In reverent memory
of Master Kung Wei (1910–1997)

*By the Sea of Java
dwelt a living dragon.*

*Oh Kung Wei,
Your kung fu, healing the poor,
Within "rusty iron" is pure steel.*

*The poor and destitute stood at your door,
Hands seeking your hands.
I brought you only apples,
You gave me three bright star gods.*

*Oh Kung Wei,
All my efforts seem to fade,
As your ease and merits shine on.*

*Even the gods have to lower
their heads to a true man.*

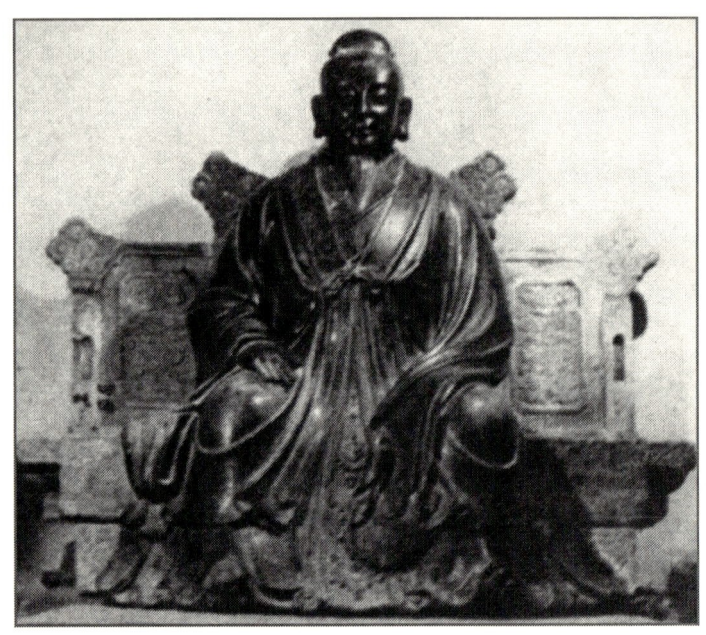

**The Immortal Ancestor Zhang Sanfeng
Founder of Taijiquan**

(A statue in his honor at Wu-Dang Temple,
Wu-Dang Mountain, Hubei Province, China)

Preface

This particular work on the Chen Kung Series was in dire need of revision. By restructuring it, including the original illustrations, adding more commentary and Chinese ideograms, this book has been greatly improved from prior versions. This book, more than any I have translated and commented on, has been a work in progress. In the Chinese text there is much assumed knowledge of the reader, and for the Chinese reader this is appropriate, but for the English reader much was needed in the way of explanation.

Over the years, a great interest in Neidan (the internal alchemy practices of Daoism) has developed, and many books have been published on the subject. This delights me, as internal alchemy is one of my main interests and practices. This book, in every sense, teaches internal alchemy, as Taijiquan is precisely internal alchemy in motion. Likewise, the Taiji Qigong Form is the very foundation for the internal alchemy aspects in the practice of Taijiquan.

As the reader will discover, for such a simple exercise it has an incredible depth, both in the internal and external sense.

It is my hope this work serves the reader well and that they partake in this practice of Taiji Qigong to improve not only their health and longevity, but the attainment of immortality as well.

Stuart Alve Olson
Winter, 2013

Acknowledgments

First, I must thank Master Chen Kung, the author of the Chinese language work. Without his diligent efforts in publishing the original Yang family documents in Shanghai, China, the Taijiquan community would sorely be missing crucial literature. Everyone involved in Taijiquan, and mostly myself, owe Mr. Chen and the Yang family a great deal of gratitude for preserving all these wonderful documents. In 2004, I corresponded with Chen Kung's grandson, Donald Chen. He confirmed the story of how his grandfather obtained the Yang family records, and that he had become a doctor of Chinese medicine. Chen had written two additional unpublished works on Taijiquan.

More than 25 years have passed since I first published the original version of this book, *Cultivating the Ch'i*, and I would never have attempted writing that version without the many years of instruction and help from my teacher, the late Taijiquan Master T.T. Liang. My translation work began in 1982 when he first introduced me to this material by giving me a Chinese original of the text, and encouraged me to translate it into English. Since then I have, as Liang admonished me, "incessantly mugged and bugged him" about various aspects of this work. I am very fortunate to have had him, of all the Taijiquan experts in the world, to help me along with this project. I managed only to get a droplet of his art, but I will forever be in his debt for his frustrated attempts to help me understand things beyond mere understanding. I doubt very much that I have done real justice to what we had discussed over the years, so any omissions or mistakes are mine and mine alone.

Very special thanks to my late friend from Semarang, Indonesia, Master Kung Wei, for making clear the distinctions of Qi (vital breath energy) and Jin (sinew intrinsic energy). His knowledge of these subjects was truly deep and profound. I will forever be in his debt, and I miss him deeply.

Vern Peterson for all his initial support of this work and friendship; Dan Miller for providing the rare photographs of Yang Luchan and Yang Banhou. Much appreciation is due to Patrick Gross without whom this book would not exist in its present condition. He spent many hours reorganizing the entire material, as well as designing and laying out this new edition.

Finally, many thanks to all my students and friends, who through their support and diligent efforts, have been a source of inspiration for me. To all of them and to the others mentioned above, I bow in deep respect and gratitude.

—*Stuart Alve Olson*

Contents

Preface vii
Acknowledgements viii
Zhang Sanfeng xii
Yang Family Lineage xiv
Master Chen Kung xv

Introduction 1
    Taiji Qi (Qigong Methods for Developing Internal Energy) 5

Chapter One: Nourishing Life 9
    Regarding the Martial Arts 11
    Inherited and Cultivated Qi 15
    Reasons for Nourishing-Life 17

Chapter Two: Mind-Intent and Qi 21
    Qi and the Mind 21
    Regarding the Martial Arts 28
    Verses on Qi 29

Chapter Three: Mobilizing the Qi 32
    Moving the Qi 37
    Heng and Ha 39
        Methods of Qigong Breathing 41

Chapter Four: Taiji Qigong 47
    Procedures for Strengthening and Mobilizing Qi 47
    Taijiquan Qigong Exercise 51

Chapter Five: **Qigong Stances** 89
    Expressing the Qi 91
    Post Stances 94
        Riding a Horse Stance 95
        Chuan Zi Stances 96
    Cai Tui Exercise 100

Chapter Six: **Meditation** 104
    Civil and Martial Cultivation 106
    Seated Meditation Qigong 108
    Four Methods of Circulating Qi 114
        Method One: Circuit for After Heaven Breathing 118
        Method Two: Circuit for Before Heaven Breathing 120
        Method Three: Lesser Heavenly Circuits 122
        Method Four: Greater Heavenly Circuit 125
    Concluding Comments 128

About Stuart Alve Olson 131
Suggested Reading 134
About the Sanctuary of Dao 136

Zhang Sanfeng

Song Dynasty Immortal Ancestor and Founder of Taijiquan

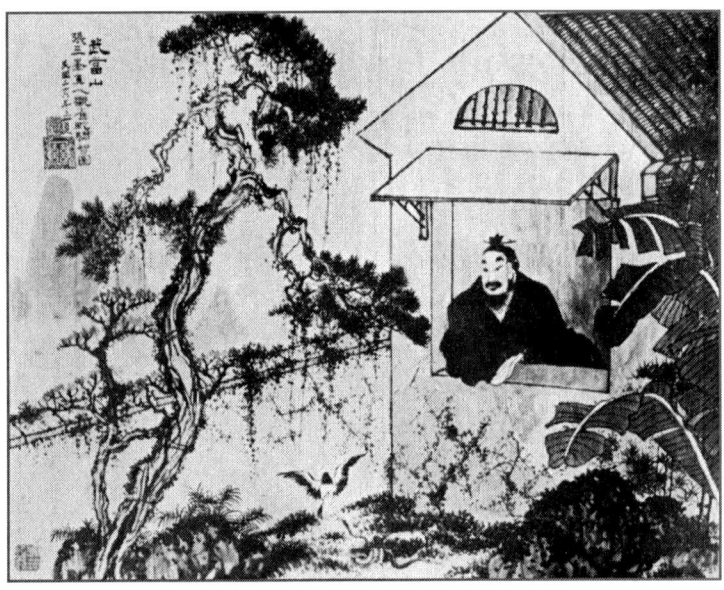

Painting of Zhang Sanfeng watching a bird attacking a snake from his meditation hut on Wu-Dang Mountain, Hubei Province.

From the simple event of watching a bird attacking a snake, Master Zhang formulated the basic premises for the practice of Taijiquan.

As the snake evaded the strikes of the bird's beak and wings, Master Zhang noticed that it would coil and twist away when attacked. When the bird struck the snake's tail, the snake's head would immediately respond. If the bird then attacked the head, the snake's tail would respond. And when the bird resorted to assaulting the snake's body, its head and tail both responded.

After several failed attempts to defeat the snake, the bird surrendered and flew away.

From observing the snake, Zhang concluded that employing the entire body as one unit was more powerful than just moving the arms or legs independently, being pliable and relaxed meant greater efficiency and endurance of movement, and that the yielding can overcome the unyielding.

From the insights acquired in watching the bird and snake, Zhang was inspired to create the Thirteen Postures of Taijiquan.

Zhang Sanfeng is also credited with writing the *Tai Ji Quan Treatise* (太極拳論, *Tai Ji Quan Lun*,* and *Tai Ji Secret Arts of Refining the Elixir of Immortality* (太極煉丹秘訣, *Tai Ji Lian Dan Bi Jue)*. This later book is one of the best internal alchemy works in Chinese, wherein his meditation methods, especially, are very effective and adaptable to modern culture.

---

* See my book *Tai Ji Quan Treatise,* Valley Spirit Arts, 2012 for a fuller biography of Zhang Sanfeng and translation of this text.

Yang Family Lineage
Yang Style Founder, Yang Luchan
陽露禪
(1799–1872)

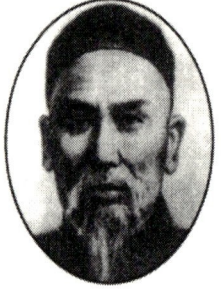

Yang Banhou
陽班侯
(1837–1892)
Son of Yang Luchan

Yang Jianhou
陽健侯
(1842–1917)
Son of Yang Luchan

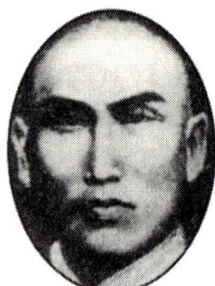

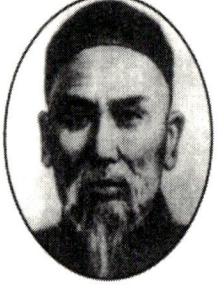

Yang Shaohou
陽少侯
(1862–1930)
Son of Jianhou

Yang Chengfu
陽澄甫
(1883–1936)
Son of Jianhou

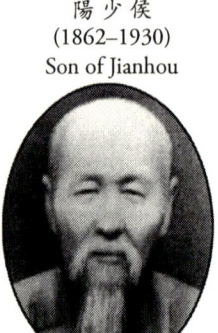

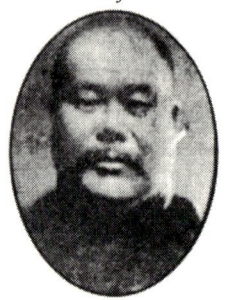

Master Chen Kung

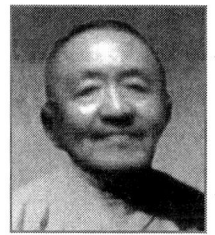

Born in 1906, Master Chen Kung—a.k.a., Yearning K. Chen and Chen Yen-lin—passed away in Shanghai, China, in 1980. His book *Tai Ji Quan Sword, Saber, Staff, and Dispersing-Hands Combined* revolutionized many aspects of Taijiquan practice and theory, especially those concerning his discourses on Intrinsic Energy (勁, Jin), Sensing-Hands (推手, Tui-Shou), Greater Rolling-Back (大攄, Da-Lu), and Dispersing-Hands (散手, San-Shou). His explanations of intrinsic energies (Jin) had never before appeared in any previous Taijiquan-related book, which really made him and his work an enigma. In 1978, Master Jou Tsung-hwa met with him in Shanghai and reported that Chen started practicing Taijiquan at age four and was a doctor of Chinese medicine.

Around 1930, Chen Kung, a rich merchant and student of Yang Chengfu (陽澄甫) asked to borrow the family transcripts for just one evening so that he might read them to enhance his practice. Chen had been a loyal and dedicated student, so Yang Chengfu consented, knowing that in one night it would be difficult for even a fast reader to finish the book. What Yang didn't know was that Chen had hired seven transcribers to work through the night to copy the entire work. After his disappearance (around 1932) he changed professions from merchant to doctor of Chinese medicine. During that year portions of the manuscript started appearing in various journals, which infuriated the Yang family.

Later, in 1943, Chen's entire copied notes appeared in book form and enjoyed rapid sales throughout China. This further infuriated the Yang family, who then released their own book claiming that Chen's publication was a forgery and that their new, smaller work was the genuine material. Chen, in typical Chinese style, claimed his book contained his own theories and that he only used the Yang family name for authenticity. This was Chinese politics at its best.

Master Liang told me this story. He had heard it through his teacher Prof. Cheng Man-ch'ing who heard it from his teacher, Yang Chengfu. With this kind of oral testimony I was never sure about the details. However, Master Jou Tsung-hwa said that Chen Kung confirmed the story when they met in 1978, and now Donald Chen, Chen Kung's grandson, confirmed it to me as well.

Before anyone accuses Chen of any wrongdoing, clearly the Taijiquan world owes him a great debt, whatever the ethics or politics that were involved. The Yang family teachings might well have remained hidden or become lost; likewise, the Yang family might never have published the various works of their own. An even greater result was that many masters, for whatever reasons, began publishing their works as well. Chen's courage created a chain reaction of teachers going public with their knowledge.

In 1947, Chen Kung's, *Tai Chi Ch'uan: Its Effects and Practical Applications,* appeared from Willow Pattern Press in Shanghai, China. The book lists Yearning K. Chen as the author and Kuo Shuichang as the translator. The interesting thing about this book is that it doesn't appear to be wholly derived from the original 1943 Chinese version of Chen Kung's work used with this present translation. The chapters on physics, psychology, and morality included in the English edition make it completely distinct from the text I used for this work. The solo form instructions and practical application explanations are similar to the 1943 Chinese text, but the two are not identical by any other means, and it did not include the discourses on Taiji Qigong as presented here.

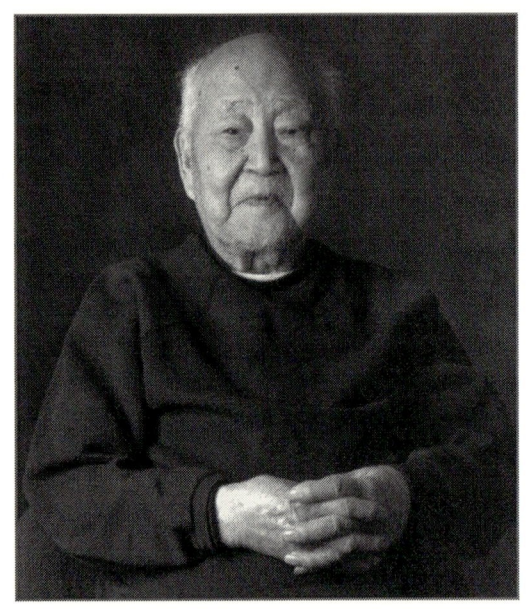

"Chen Kung's book is without doubt second to none on the subject of Taijiquan."

Master T.T. Liang
梁東材太極拳師
(1900 to 2002)

Introduction

The genius of Master Yang Luchan, founder of the Yang family system of Taijiquan, has yet to be fully appreciated and investigated. These translations and writings will hopefully provide a big step in that direction. I say this because having intensively investigated the original Chinese book from Chen Kung, it immediately dawned on me how incredibly ingenious Yang Luchan's manner of teaching was. No other system of Taijiquan is as precise nor as complete as the style Yang created. Every method of training was developed to focus on one aspect of Taijiquan and yet overlap with all the other training methods. Whether it be the Qigong training or the intrinsic energy methods, all are designed to draw out certain internal and external skills of the practicer.

The Two Primary Energy Skills Trained in Taijiquan
— Qi and Jin —

氣

Qi: Breath, Vital-Life Energy, Internal Heat, Steam-like Vapor for Mobilization of Blood, Internal Power, an Inherent Oxygen in the Blood, and Externally Expressed Power.

Jin: Intrinsic Energy, Relaxed and Alert Sensitivity, Power of the Sinews and Tendons, Whip-like Energy, Nimbleness and Lightness of the Body, Energy of the Entire Body Used as One Unit

This book may seem a little overwhelming when first reading it. My advice is to go slow, reread the material as many times as possible, and gradually absorb the information. Sometimes we take in too much information too quickly and so walk away with nothing. The material is intensive and extensive, and will take time to digest. Although it presents the basic, foundational information for developing internal energy, full understanding of the book may only come to those who have succeeded in attaining higher levels of Taijiquan. But do not be disheartened, because Taijiquan internal skills can be acquired by anyone who invests time and patience.

Presenting this book has been exciting and humbling. It is hard for a writer/translator to provide a publication that can possibly bring more light and clarity to a subject that has already been clouded with way too much mystification. As I said before, the content of this particular volume, I think, is a milestone within the available literature on Taijiquan, especially in light of the additions and changes made to it since I first published the work in 1986. Chen Kung's book has, of course, been available to the Chinese reader for over seventy years, and there is no question about how much has been quietly borrowed from it by Taijiquan authors and teachers. So it is really an honor to be presenting (once again) this translation on the subject of Taiji Qigong.

The idea of internal energy (Qi) associated with Taijiquan has for a number of years bordered on the mystical, and indeed at very high levels of the art this can be true, but the mainstream of Taijiquan skills are quite available to anyone, providing they practice correctly, study well, and seek out reputable teachers. This work, in my opinion, provides many details of correct practice, and adds much in the way of clarifying Taijiquan functional theory.

This book covers a broad field of Taijiquan theory and practice. I found myself in the dilemma of how much to comment on. In reality, each paragraph, and in some cases each sentence, deserves lengthy commentary. The problem in doing this is repetition of fundamentals, as everything that is theoretical here interrelates with everything that is practical, much like the familiar problem of discussing chickens but forever backtracking to discuss the formation of the egg. The translated text and commentary function as a whole, however, if one remembers that nothing here is isolated from the principles of Taijiquan. The material should be read many times to assure that you retain as much of the information as possible.

The main emphasis of this book is to provide the preliminary foundations for the practice of Taijiquan, namely "Qigong." Ideally, anyone beginning their Taijiquan career would begin with the fundamental exercises explained in this book.

The majority of practicers who seek to master Taijiquan have to more or less backtrack in their studies, normally first learning the solo form postures and then later seeking out the fundamental exercises and principles of the Qigong aspects. It would do well for the Taijiquan community to consider this problem carefully. If we ask, "How many Taijiquan practicers really understand, or can actually apply, the absolute and necessary fundamentals of Song (鬆, relaxed alertness and non-muscular exertion), the One-Breath (一氣, Yi Qi), Mind-Intent (意, Yi), Sinking the Qi into the Dan-Tian (氣沉丹田, Qi Zhen Dan Tian), Abiding by the Dan-Tian (住丹田, Zhu Dan Tian), or Adhering the Qi to the Spine (氣貼脊背, Qi Tie Ji Bei)?" the answer would be very few—infinitesimally few. Knowing what is required for true mastery of the art, and the sheer lack of actual masters, we must also ask, "How much of the Taijiquan currently being taught and practiced is really Taijiquan?"

Too often Taijiquan is practiced and viewed as just some sort of external gymnastic for improving health, but Taijiquan is predominantly an internal art (內丹, Neidan). Fundamentally, it is internal alchemy in motion. Ideally, in practice only 10 percent of the movement is expressed externally; 90 percent is unseen and sensed internally. The great Taijiquan Master Yang Chengfu stated, *"Taijiquan is meditation in action, and activity within meditation."* Alertness of non-muscular exertion, the One-Breath, Mind-Intent, Sinking Qi into the Dan-Tian, Abiding by the Dan-Tian, and Adhering Qi to the Spine are not external activities—they are purely internal. Therefore, a physically expanded and gracious appearing display of Taijiquan movement is not necessarily good, effective, or true internalized Taijiquan.

None of what I'm saying is meant to imply that just learning Taijiquan without delving into the fundamentals and principles of this work is useless. I, as well as the majority of Taijiquan practicers, started out by learning just the Taijiquan postures, and I cannot deny the many health benefits I acquired from that initial external practice. But, I can honestly say, without question, it wasn't until I underwent this backtracking into the Qigong aspects of Taijiquan that I began realizing real progress internally. To fully understand and master Taijiquan it must be internalized, and this only occurs through the practice and adherence to its fundamental energies. Therefore, the principles and exercises presented in this book are essential to the mastery of internalizing Taijiquan.

Taiji Qi (Qigong Methods for Developing Internal Energy)
Qigong means, "the skill of breath/Qi" or "to work the breath/Qi." In the Chinese language the term *Qi* has several layers of meaning. First is breath, the very function which animates the human body. Qi, derived from the inhalation and exhalation of breath, is like a latent oxygen within the blood and body, much the same as steam is latent within water. Water and steam are essentially the same, as are breath and Qi. Just as steam can be turned into a very powerful energy, the same is true of Qi. *Gong* means, "skill," "work," or "effort," the same Chinese character used in the more popular term *kung-fu* (gong-fu).

The most important aspect of experiencing Qi revolves around a Qi cavity (or center) in the lower abdomen called the Dan-Tian (Field of Elixir). It is in essence a person's very center of being. In Qigong practice—as well as in meditation, martial arts, yoga, and all spiritual practices—the Dan-Tian is the very source from which Qi is first accumulated and mobilized within the body. Every exercise shown in this book relies heavily on the idea that the Dan-Tian is not only being paid attention to, but that it is intrinsically sensed by the practicer. This cannot be overstated, nothing in the way of Qi experience will occur unless absolute focus is put on the Dan-Tian.

When Qi begins to accumulate in the lower abdomen, and specifically in the Dan-Tian, it will produce actual physical effects. The location of this Qi cavity is 3 inches behind your navel. The more the breath is worked properly, the more Qi from that breath begins accumulating in the Dan-Tian. From this accumulation, the Qi can be willed to move from the Dan-Tian and through the various Qi meridians of the body, where it will begin concentrating within other Qi cavities of the body. It is creating this movement, or mobilization, of Qi that is called Qigong.

The *Taiji 21-Posture Qigong Form* is the focal exercise of this work, concentrating on the learning of mobilizing external physical movement from breath, Qi, and Mind-Intent. Experiencing this internal means of mobilizing movement is usually a major breakthrough for most Taijiquan students, as the majority of beginners just use muscular exertion to move their arms. However, in this exercise the arms, after continuous practice, attain the sensation of floating throughout the movements of the form.

There are two ways in which to get a sense of what this floating of the arms feels like without ever having done Taijiquan or Qigong. The first is to stand upright and relaxed, with hands and arms placed in front of the thighs. Put all your attention into your lower abdomen and just feel and sense the breath expanding and contracting the abdomen. Gradually as you do this you will feel your hands and arms floating upward, without the use of any muscular force.

The second manner is to stand in a doorway, place both palms on the inside of the door jams and press the hands as hard as you can outward for fifteen seconds or so. After withdrawing from the door jams your hands and arms will rise upward, again without any muscular actions needed. This is purely the reaction of Qi and blood rushing back into the arms. So it is this type of sensation, floating of the hands and arms, that is experienced and developed in both Qigong and Taijiquan.

The processes for developing Qi, to actually feel it in the body, starts with the breath itself. Breath is naturally warm and from concentrating the warm breath in the lower abdomen (Dan-Tian) the blood and other body fluids are likewise warmed. The warmed blood then circulates more efficiently through the muscles and tendons of the body. As this increased circulation of warm blood occurs in the muscles, the heat (炁, Qi)[1] then begins penetrating the bones and increases the marrow content of them. Thus making the person stronger and more pliable, as well as bringing about youthfulness to their entire body and being.

1. There are two Chinese characters used in the explanation of Qigong, and both translate as Qi. The first character 氣 is a reference to the vapor-like sensations created internally, and to the sense of a power deriving from the Dan-Tian. The second Qi character, 炁, is used almost exclusively concerning the heat in the body produced from abdominal breathing.

This process of developing Qi is normally referred to as Free Circulation of Qi (自如氣周, Zi Ru Qi Zhou) and is stimulated primarily through specific body posturing and movement and keeping the breath low in the abdomen. Simultaneously, however, because of the concentration of the breath low in the abdomen, the Qi will begin accumulating (積氣, Ji Qi) in the Dan-Tian and will begin expanding, making the Dan-Tian evermore substantial and real to the practicer. It is the realization of these two effects, *Free Circulation of Qi* and *Accumulation of Qi,* that are the primary and specific goals of Taiji Qigong and all the Taijiquan practices as well. Taijiquan has two major divisions of training, the development of Qi and the development of Jin (intrinsic energies—for use in self-defense).

Beyond these two goals of Free Circulation of Qi and Accumulating Qi, the higher and deeper processes of Daoist alchemy (內丹, Neidan, literally "internal elixir") then come into play, namely circulating the Qi in and through the eight major subtle Qi meridians of the body for refinement into the elixir of immortality. But, to do this there must first be sufficient Qi in the Dan-Tian in which to mobilize, hence the usefulness and purpose of Taiji Qigong.

Many students over the years have adamantly praised the short, powerful Qigong exercise presented in this book. I don't think it wise, however, to promise too much in the way of Qi development to those who only read this book and make a half-hearted effort at practicing the methods. The exercises require continued and daily practice over a long time. Without sustained effort it is doubtful anyone could derive the full benefits of these exercises. Like any art form, the keys to successful realization of skills lie in perseverance and repetitive practice.

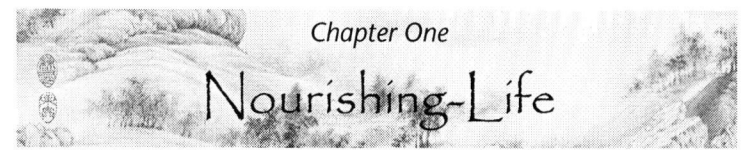

Chapter One
Nourishing-Life

養生

[Author's Commentary]

The purpose of this chapter in Chen Kung's book is mainly to encourage people to practice any of the exercises of Taijiquan so they might enjoy a healthy life even in old age. The material covers a wide range of concepts associated with the practice of Taijiquan, all of which provide what Daoists term Yang Sheng (養生), or "Nourishing-Life."

[Chen Kung's Text]

"All the practices of the Taijiquan system are vehicles in themselves for refining and disciplining the completion of Nourishing-Life. You can mobilize and stimulate the Spirit of Vitality, which will feel like flowing water through the meridians of your body, rather than stagnant water you cannot feel move. This is like the analogy of a door pivot, which never becomes worm-eaten.

> The essential purpose of Daoist Nourishing Life practices is to develop the Jing (精, essence), Qi (氣, breath-vitality), and Shen (神, spirit)—collectively referred to as the Three Treasures (三寶, San Bao). This process is also called Guarding the One (守一, Shou Yi) or Abiding by the Dan-Tian (住丹田, Zhu Dan Tian), which are accomplished through Mind-Intent and Qi.

Nourishing-Life commonly means "to create life," but in Daoism it is a generic term denoting the idea of cultivating the Three Treasures. More often, Nourishing-Life is a reference made just to the hygiene practices of Daoism, such as Taijiquan, Qigong, and meditation. However, in a fuller Daoist definition, Nourishing-Life is divided into eight branches of practice:

1. Tranquil Sitting (靜坐, Jing Zuo)
2. Guiding and Enticing (導引, Dao Yin)
3. Purifying Breath (吐納, Tu Na)
4. Ingesting Medicines (服藥, Fu Yao)
5. Conserving Qi (覆氣, Fu Qi)
6. Refining Qi (煉氣, Lian Qi)
7. Abstaining from Grains (辟谷, Bi Gu)
8. Bedchamber Arts (房中術, Fang Zhong Shu)

An ancient Daoist ode on Nourishing-Life reads:
 "Hearing the sound of flowing water nourishes the ears;
 "Seeing the green of trees and plants nourishes the eyes;
 "Studying books that explain principles nourishes the mind;
 "Playing the lute and practicing writing nourishes the fingers;
 "Wandering about on foot with a staff nourishes the feet;
 "Tranquility of mind and sitting in meditation nourishes
     the nature;
 "Harmonizing the Qi nourishes the muscles and tendons."

You can use any of the Taijiquan training exercises as a vehicle for Nourishing-Life—the Taijiquan solo form, Qigong, the two-person training methods, sword, saber, or staff.

The "Spirit of Vitality" (精神, Jing Shen) is a term for the refined essences of the Three Treasures (Jing, Qi, and Shen), which in simpler terms is the Qi made capable of moving through the meridians of the body because of its stimulation from Nourishing-Life practices.

In Daoism, to "refine and discipline" your body is called Duan Lian (鍛煉). *Duan* means to "forge metal," hence the idea of discipline. *Lian* means to "smelt," thus the notion of refinement. Daoists normally use this metallurgical analogy of forging and smelting raw ore to acquire pure steel as a way to explain the internal alchemical process. Hence, in Daoism, the idea is to first discipline the Jing (forge the raw ore), then refine the Qi (smelt into iron), and in the end obtain pure Shen (refine into pure steel).

Regarding the Martial Arts

"There are numerous styles of Chinese boxing, some with very ancient histories and origins. Regarding external appearances, there are those styles which favor hard techniques and those which favor softer ones.

"Different generations have regarded Shaolin Kung Fu (少林功夫) energies as mere external displays, emphasizing only the unyielding; they likewise regard Taijiquan self-defense energies as only a collection of internal imaginings, emphasizing only that which is yielding. They do not understand that the highest skills of Shaolin and Taijiquan are the combination of the unyielding and the yielding."

Shaolin starts with the unyielding, and Taijiquan with the yielding. Yet both seek the state of effortlessness created by Shen Ming (神明, Illuminated Spirit), and natural, spontaneous responses. Even though both schools develop the martial skills of intrinsic energies, Shaolin relies more heavily on developing

Li (external strength), whereas Taijiquan focuses on energy developing out of *Jin*[1] (internal power). In analogy, external strength is like the energy coming from a moving stick, and internal power like the energy coming from a whip.

1. See *Tai Ji Jin—The Intrinsic Energies of Taijiquan* by Stuart Alve Olson. *Chen Kung Series: From the Secret Records of Yang Luchan,* Valley Spirit Arts, 2013.

"An error that occurs, however, with those who favor only hard styles is that the feet and legs lean in all the movements; they do not realize that leaning will obstruct the Qi. Taijiquan primarily develops soft skin and flesh; the skin and flesh are soft like cotton, yet the internal Qi is strong, like iron of superior quality. This is called, 'an iron bar wrapped in silk or cotton.'"

Leaning during the practice of Taijiquan movements is avoided because it creates an extreme bending and stress of the joints from the waist down, which causes obstruction of blood flow and Qi. In Taijiquan, it is very important not to allow the knee of the front leg to go past the toes, so if looking down you should still be able to see the toes of the foot. Otherwise, the knee has been bent too far forward and the weight cannot be displaced evenly in the foot. This not only obstructs the circulation of blood and Qi, but deadens the ability for issuing the intrinsic energy (Jin).

The notion of the arm feeling like "an iron bar wrapped in cotton" is a result of the Qi penetrating into the bone, turning it into marrow (the iron bar), and the effect of Song energy on the muscles, sinews, and tendons (silk or cotton).

"It is really immaterial what school or style you practice, as you should not give undue attention to either hardness or softness. Just make sure the main principles are not neglected, even momentarily. Focus entirely on whatever vehicle is being made use of to acquire skill.

"When practicing Taijiquan, you may form the habit of being too soft and yielding [in which case you become lethargic and sluggish]. There really is no advantage in this. Students should always be conscious to the advantages of fundamental principles, which are: practicing the movements slowly and evenly, inhaling and exhaling naturally to accumulate Qi and concentrate the Shen, and never employing muscular strength (Li) too excessively. It is through softness and gentleness that you achieve mastery. This softness and gentleness means soft and continuous movements in conjunction with harmonious breathing.

"Jing, Qi, and Shen [the Three Treasures] and all the intrinsic energies ideally should be developed to their fullest capacity. Neither the internal nor external aspects of these energies should be based entirely on the kind of softness and gentleness that leads to lethargy or immobility. This is central to Sensing-Hands (推手, Tui-Shou) practices. When brute-force (拙力, Zhuo-Li) is too strong, it cannot exist for long; and likewise intrinsic energy cannot be totally devoid of strength either."

> Becoming too soft and yielding means becoming so relaxed that you are in a state of collapse. Taijiquan is an external appearance of relaxation, but internally there is an alert vitality. In the case of brute-force it literally means, "clumsy and unskilled strength." Taijiquan, however, makes use of both Li (strength) and Jin (intrinsic energy). Probably the best analogy for this can be seen in how a gorilla uses its

strength. It is surprising to see how relaxed a gorilla's muscles are when climbing or even fighting. Even though gorillas have great strength, they rarely express any muscular tension or strain in their movements.

"Consider the expression 'Removing one thousand catties with only four ounces.' This is to have the Skillful Energy (巧勁, Qiao Jin) of four ounces. Attempting to remove one thousand catties with only brute-force (clumsy and undisciplined strength) [and] without the intrinsic energy of four ounces is impossible. How can this be done?"

This "four ounces of Skillful Energy" can be seen in an example of some large, heavy object attached to a rope swinging down toward someone. In this case, if the person were to simply use the waist by turning to the side and away from the object, and simultaneously attach their hand lightly to the side of the object, the object can be directed away without causing injury. It is the lightly attaching of the hand that is referred to as "four ounces of strength." The same idea applies to an incoming punch, kick, or attack from an opponent.

"Through slowness you can later be soft; through evenness you can be gentle. The capability of being soft and gentle will cause the muscle and bone to open. The Qi and blood will circulate harmoniously. From this the breath will become deep and long and the Spirit of Vitality can be stimulated and brought forth.

"If you suffer in old age from such serious illnesses as consumption, heart disease, high blood pressure, or numbness in the extremities, you should take up these exercises."

Inherited and Cultivated Qi

"By practicing Taijiquan you can completely cure the insufficiencies of the Before Heaven (inherited from parents) and repair the injuries of the After Heaven (acquired from our own physical self-abuses). So, if possible, when you are still young and able bodied enough, you should devote yourself entirely to continuous practice, without interruption. As a result you will obtain not only a lifetime of benefit, but a life worth writing about."

Before Heaven (先天, Xian Tian) and *After Heaven* (後天, Hou Tian) are Daoist concepts expressing many aspects of self-cultivation and philosophy. Normally, and here in the text, it refers to the quality of Qi (from insufficient to abundant) that you inherited from your parents (Before Heaven), and to the dissipation of Qi you experience from self-abuses or to the increased Qi you develop and acquire from Nourishing-Life practices (After Heaven).

The philosophy of Before and After Heaven is very broad and abstruse, equal to that of Five-Element theory and Yin-Yang theory—all of which interconnect and, for the most part, form the basis of Chinese philosophy.

Insufficiency of the Before Heaven means that a person was not born with sufficient Jing, Qi, or Shen, and therefore suffers physically or mentally in one form or another.

Repair the injuries of the After Heaven means to cure or eliminate problems we inflicted upon ourselves through physical and mental self-abuses. As examples, we might have had bad eating habits or unduly placed stresses in our life. So *repair* would mean to take up good eating habits and eliminate the stress responses. Therefore, *"curing the insufficiencies and repairing the injuries"* is a reference directed at taking up the practices of Taijiquan, Qigong, or meditation—or any of the eight branches of Nourishing-Life practices for that matter.

Other examples of Before and After Heaven interpretations:

Before Heaven represents inhalation, and After Heaven, exhalation.

Before Heaven is the Qi ascending the spine; After Heaven is the Qi descending on the front of the body.

Before Heaven is associated with "Embryonic Breathing" and After Heaven with "Natural Breathing."

Some books refer to Before and After Heaven as Prenatal Breath (先天氣, Xian Tian Qi) and Postnatal Breath *(*後天氣, Hou Tian Qi).

The Eight Diagrams, or trigrams, (八卦圖, Ba Gua Tu) appear in Before Heaven and After Heaven arrangements.

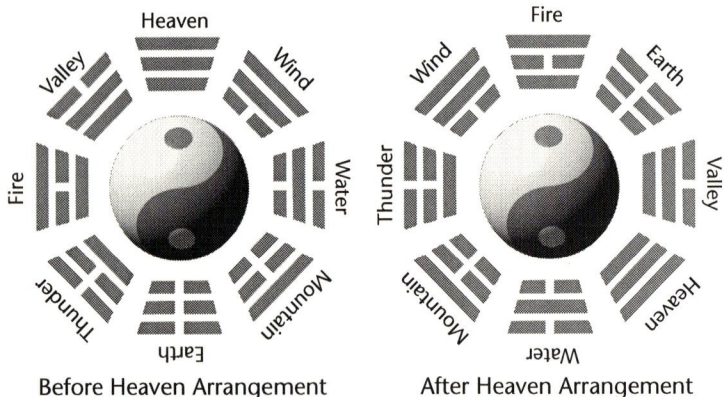

Before Heaven Arrangement　　　After Heaven Arrangement

Reasons for Nourishing-Life
"During your youth, the stamina is more than sufficient to handle strenuous work and to accomplish tasks with relative speed. If you become physically vigorous and robust by practicing Taijiquan in the years that you are naturally able bodied, then in old age you can succeed in illuminating your spirit and in the completion of bright Qi. Every movement will be light and nimble, there will be no affliction of the waist and no back pain, no withering of the Spirit of Vitality, or anxious breathing and groaning, which are all symptoms of disease."

Sufficient vigor and stamina here is a direct reference to that period, especially in young males when the sexual energy has not yet been damaged through long term or excessive dissipation of semen. In women, the same damage occurs over time because of the menstrual cycle. Men who can conserve their sexual energy and women who can lessen their menstrual flow will in old age be free of many of the ills of aging.

"These types of conditions are quite similar to that of saving money, because in our youth we can also save our bodies through discipline and refinement, like a daily accumulation of virtue. Then in old age we can enjoy and use this. Daily accumulation is of no further concern. Otherwise in a moment of crisis there is nothing to fall back on. People of different generations have not really understood this viewpoint. For the most part, there are two views concerning this matter:
1) During youth the energy is strong and the body does not normally suffer many illnesses. During youth we still have stamina and the sexual energy [精, Jing] is not yet damaged

or injured through excessive dissipation, still having sufficient physical and mental strength. So we don't worry about strengthening the Qi or Spirit of Vitality.
2) Then there are those who practice these exercises for just a period of time and then think they can dispense with their practice, but in their old age as they approach death they suffer bitterly because they no longer practice.

"How can anyone possibly know beforehand that these two viewpoints are utterly erroneous? Because young people have strong and vital bodies, with the Qi functioning more than satisfactorily, they certainly do not see the beneficial outcome of disciplining and refining the body and mind. When reaching old age, on the other hand, the Qi weakens. At this time, to your regret, your resistance is not sufficient internally, and you suffer when you reach the point of death. The experience of those who practice these exercises and have these conditions will be exactly the opposite.

"Taijiquan bases itself exclusively on gentleness, softness, naturalness, and bringing you back to your original nature. Daily practice makes the muscles and bones softer and more pliable, and it especially causes the breath to become natural. These are the results of disciplining and refining the Jing, Qi, and Shen to the end of your days. How then can you consider dispensing with your exercise or wish to suffer bitterly?

"The old masters of Taijiquan, in days gone by, would very often sit cross-legged, smile, and then pass away. This is evidence that they found the two previous viewpoints to be erroneous. For others who practice Taijiquan it would be satisfying enough to just attain a peaceful death.

"When practicing the postures of Taijiquan you should seek to be correct and not rely on brute-force. You must be centered, calm, and composed.

"Embracing the Origin and Guarding the One, without thought and without anxiety. Take every opportunity to practice."

> *Embracing the Origin* (抱元, Bao Yuan) and *Guarding the One* (守一, Shou Yi) mean the same thing. They are the very essence of all Daoist self-cultivation practices. In Taijiquan specifically they are identical to the meaning and practice of "to abide by the Dan-Tian" or "sink the Qi into the Dan-Tian."
>
> In the practice of Taijiquan, and all the practices associated with it, "abiding by the Dan-Tian" or "sinking the Qi into the Dan-Tian" is absolutely crucial if any progress or mastery is to be attained.

"Pay attention and make the entire body comfortable. If, after a while you become weary, rest. Should the practice periods be long or short? Who can know completely each individual's energy? It is not necessary to be too ambitious or too tied to old conventions concerning practice. But those who do constantly practice can endure because they hold it in such high esteem. If this is the case and you are able to train constantly, then eventually you will certainly acquire the benefits of practice.

"In the beginning of your practice, you may not have the necessary motivation to really work the blood and Qi, but in the blink of an eye the flag is seen and the entire interior is strengthened. The Qi will function fully, the 'hundred illnesses' will be eliminated and vitality and health preserved intact."

When *"the flag is seen"* is an analogy taken from *The Mental Elucidation of the Thirteen Kinetic Postures* (十三勢行功心, Shi San Shi Xing Gong Xin), a Taijiquan treatise attributed to the immortal Wang Zongyue (王宗岳) of the Ming Dynasty. It says: *"The mind is the commander; the Qi is the flag; the waist is the banner."* So, seeing the flag (banner) means that you realize and experience the Qi. You will then want to completely devote yourself to practice.

"In the blink of an eye" means that at some point in your practice the Qi will just appear—as if out of nowhere. In my own case this happened one evening while practicing Taijiquan with Master Liang. The sensation was several things simultaneously. There was this immediate surge of energy coming from my lower abdomen, moving up my spine, and then out my hands and arms. No experience in my life ever gave me the sensation of such overwhelming strength as this did. I remember thinking that I could uproot a tree if I had wanted too. Just after the sensation left my hands and arms, I stopped and stood there looking at the palms of my hands in amazement. Master Liang also stopped. He looked at me with a happy grin and said, "This is called 'unconscious movement of Qi.' Your work now is to make that happen consciously whenever you want to."

"Therefore, seek out the Way of Nourishing-Life with the practice of this orthodox art of Taijiquan. But above all rely upon your own self to generate effective results."

Chapter Two
Mind-Intent and Qi

意 氣

The most important piece of information being related here is that Mind-Intent and Qi are mutually interdependent. This is a point well explained in this chapter. Indeed, on the level of importance, this chapter outweighs the rest. Too many people practice Taijiquan with the idea that just breathing low in the abdomen will somehow produce Qi. The practitioner might gain a little benefit from this, but will certainly not achieve what is called "bright Qi." More likely they will experience the negative Qi of scorching heat.

Many ill-informed Qigong practitioners, in the East and West, have suffered the ill effects of not understanding, or not having been taught, how to properly Abide by the Dan-Tian, how to properly develop Mind-Intent, and how to internally train the One Breath. This chapter provides the correct information for these practices.

Qi and the Mind

"Within each person there is Mind-Intent and Qi, both of which are invisible and formless."

Mind-Intent—in the practice of Taijiquan, the function of the Mind-Intent (or will) is both transcendentally and intrinsically connected with Qi. Mind-Intent is neither a conditioned response nor unconscious reaction. It is a reaction founded in awareness, intuition, and sensitive alertness. Mind-Intent, however, is "conditioned" in that it is developed over a long time from the practice of various Taijiquan exercises. The Mind-Intent is also "unconscious" in that the rational thinking mind is not used. The problem in defining Mind-Intent is an empirical one in that you must first be truly capable of Sinking the Qi into the Dan-Tian, which then strengthens the vitality of Mind-Intent, which in turn will affect the mind, producing tranquility. So without initiating the use of Mind-Intent, however vague at first, to Sink the Qi into the Dan-Tian, the Mind-Intent cannot be made strong enough for you to truly realize the difference between Mind-Intent and mind.

Qi is the vital life energy and breath. There are many explanations of what Qi is, such as an inherent oxygen in the blood for stamina and vitality, or a subtle cosmic energy which constitutes life, growth, and motion in all things. Both these, and all other explanations, are primarily true. Most teachings and teachers, however, prefer to explain its stimulation, nourishment, accumulation, and/or circulation than to attempt the difficult task of defining it.

In Taijiquan and seated meditation you can experience the sensations of Qi when 1) Mind-Intent sinks the Qi into the Dan-Tian, 2) when Mind-Intent becomes vital, and 3) the mind is tranquil—then Qi will not only be sensed, but will circulate freely throughout the body.

"It is essential to know that the Qi is produced within the body to harness this energy is extremely important as the Qi and the body must satisfy each other's needs.

"In application, the Qi stimulates the blood and nourishes it. This is the process of perfecting the Qi. The heat from the Qi rises up from the Gates of Life (命門, Ming Men, kidneys). The Jing [physical vitality and sexual energy] should then be cherished and nourished. Both the Jing and Qi should be repeatedly stimulated and perfected. Daoist schools call this, *perfecting the fire and water,* or the *internal elixir.* Daoists seek to retain the Qi and store it in the Dan-Tian. They regard the Qi as being an exceptionally precious possession."

The *Gates of Life* are Qi cavities associated with the kidneys, located over each of the kidneys on each side of the spine. This location is as well where the adrenal glands reside.

Jing is usually translated as sperm (for the male) and menstrual fluids (for women). Jing, however, is not necessarily just a substance, but rather the subtle energy that produces it—i.e., sexual force or the force that gives all things form. All Daoist practices call for the conservation of Jing because it stimulates the Qi, which in turn stimulates Shen (spirit).

It should be noted that males dissipate their Jing through ejaculation of semen, and women dissipate their Jing through the menstrual flow. Hence, men need to reduce excessive dissipation and women need to reduce the flow and frequency of the menstrual blood.

Fire and Water (火水, Huo Shui) is a symbolic expression representing the interaction of Jing and Qi. The idea is that the Qi heats the Jing, which then causes both the Jing and the Qi to move. Once these move and can be circulated this is then "perfecting the fire and water." It is the heated and mobilized Jing and Qi that forms what is called the "internal elixir" (內丹, Neidan).

Field of Elixir (丹田, Dan-Tian) is the central and most important Qi center of all Chinese spiritual practices. This center, or cavity, is the source from which the Qi is stimulated and accumulated. In Taijiquan, all movement finds its source originating from the Dan-Tian. It is called the "Field of Elixir" because the Three Treasures (Jing, Qi, and Shen) are all united in this central point (Daoist analogies: pot, stove, furnace, cauldron), where they are refined to form an elixir that confers health, longevity, or immortality, depending upon the degree to which the essences of Jing, Qi, and Shen have been refined.

The process with the Dan-Tian in Taijiquan is as follows: The Mind-Intent leads the Qi down into the Dan-Tian; when this is accomplished the Qi strengthens the Mind-Intent; the more vital the Mind-Intent, the greater the mobilization of Qi and the greater the tranquility of the mind. At this point, the entire body accords with the movement of Qi guided by Mind-Intent. This is true spontaneity and Song (relaxation, alertness, and sensitivity). This is why the Taijiquan classical writings repeatedly insist on "Abiding by the Dan-Tian."

Stripping Daoism to its essentials there would be nothing left except "Abiding by the Dan-Tian" to concentrate the Jing, Qi, and Shen into this one cavity. This is the root of all Daoist philosophy and practices. Everything else is but branches and leaves. When Lao Zi (老子) says in the *Scripture on the Way and Virtue* (道德經, *Dao De Jing*), "Embracing the One (Bao Yi) and Returning to the Source (歸元, Gui Yuan)," he is saying in essence to "Abide by the Dan-Tian."

"Blood or Qi, what is to be most prized? Most people are unaware that the Qi is more substantial than the blood. The Qi acts as the master to the blood; the blood is like the assistant.

"The Qi is like the troops and the blood like the camp. During a man's entire lifetime he must depend completely upon both the troops and the camp. Supposing an army had a camp and no troops; there would then be no convoys. Likewise, having troops and no camp, there would be nowhere to unite.

"In the end, the Qi is most important and the blood is secondary. If the blood is insufficient, it is still possible to maintain life for a short period, but if the Qi is lacking, there will arise an immediate crisis, resulting in death.

"Therefore, when nourishing the Qi, what is the most important condition? Specifically, you must practice Taijiquan. Get rid of the external gymnastics. Moreover, master the production and nourishment of Qi. As the proverb says, 'Externally exercise the muscles, bones, and skin; internally train the One Breath.' Generally speaking, all of this means practicing Taijiquan."

> The *One Breath* (一口氣, Yi Kou Qi) carries various meanings ranging from connecting the inhalation and exhalation without pause, one flowing into the next; developing the mind and body unceasingly so that both function as one unit; and completion (internal attainment), which is the result of continuous repetition of practice. Sometimes this term is given as Yi Qi (one breath, one action, one energy). Here, Yi Kou Qi literally translates as "one mouthful of Qi," which in the higher practices of Daoist alchemy is a reference to the ingesting of breath or swallowing Qi—none other than what Daoists refer to as "Tortoise Breathing (龜息, Gui Xi)."

"It becomes immaterial later on whether you practice the circular motions of the solo forms, or the sparring exercises of Sensing-Hands (推手, Tui-Shou), Dispersing-Hands (散手, San-Shou, or Greater Pulling-Back (大廬, Da-Lu). All that really matters is that while performing these exercises you are conscious of breathing naturally and that your facial expression remains calm and unchanging.

"The Qi should circulate throughout the inner areas of the body. Before stretching and setting the exercise into motion, you will already be well aware of how to nourish the Qi through the exercises. The efficacy of the Taijiquan exercises is very great. So on no account corrupt your practice by training in too hasty, laborious, or fatiguing a manner. This cannot be stressed enough.

"When the blood has been completely purified, the body will become extremely strong. When the body is strong the mind is strengthened and rendered more determined. With this the spirits of Po (魄) and Hun (魂) are made strong and brave. With strong spirits you can increase your life span and benefit greatly from this longer life."

> In brief, Daoism professes that a person obtains two spirit energies at birth, the "Po" and "Hun" (Heavenly and Earthly spirits). Po represents the physical body; Hun the spiritual body. Now, at the time of death, if the Three Treasures are not cultivated, the Po descends to Earth with the Original Spirit (元神, Yuan Shen) to become a ghost, which dies off relatively quickly. If, on the other hand, the Three Treasures are cultivated, then the Original Spirit ascends to Heaven with the Hun, thus becoming one of three stages of immortal: Earthly Immortal (地仙, Di Xian), Heavenly Immortal (天仙,

Tian Xian), or Pure Yang Immortal (純陽仙, Chun Yang Xian), also called Golden Immortal (金仙, Jin Xian).

The reason for referring here to Po rather than Shen is that while alive, the Po benefits from the vitality and strength of Qi, thereby increasing the life span and enhancing the health. In Daoist alchemy there is a saying, *"Replenish the Yang with Yin."* The Po is yin, the Hun yang. Through Taijiquan practices this is exactly what occurs, yang is made strong through yin.

In the *Taijiquan Classic* it says, "From the flexible and most yielding one can become the most powerful and unyielding." So the use of Po here is symbolic of how softness and yielding can overcome the hard and unyielding, such as water wearing away at a rock, or in Lao Zi's analogy, "The tongue lasts a long time because it is soft. Because they are hard, the teeth cannot outlast the tongue."

"Students should know that the only gateway to acquiring the skills of Taijiquan is by constant cultivation of Qi. Some have said that Mind-Intent is no other than the mind (rational thinking), or that the mind is no other than the Mind-Intent. But, truly, there is both a mind and Mind-Intent; they are two separate things and should be thought of as such.

"The master of the mind is the Mind-Intent. The mind acts as only an assistant to the Mind-Intent. When the mind moves, it does so because of the Mind-Intent. When the Mind-Intent arises the Qi will follow.

"In other words: mind, Mind-Intent, and Qi are all interconnected and work in a rotational manner. When the mind is confused the Mind-Intent will disperse. When the Mind-Intent is dispersed the Qi will become insubstantial [weak].

"So it is said, 'When the Qi sinks into the Dan-Tian, the Mind-Intent is made strong and vital. With a strong and vital Mind-Intent, the mind then becomes tranquil.' Therefore, these three mutually employ each other, and in truth they must be united and not allowed to become separate.

"The application of Qi will expedite the blood circulation and stimulate the spirit. When the spirit and Qi circulation are active, they can then be put into use; otherwise, neither the Qi nor the Mind-Intent can be regulated properly."

Regarding the Martial Arts

"The way of the internal boxing arts (內拳術, Nei Quan Shu) is to have regulation without method, or principles without techniques. At some point this will be clear to the martial artist.

"Having only techniques without principles amounts to nothing more than giving up one's capital to follow an inferior scheme [to invest in a losing business venture].

"So, in the martial arts, the regulation of Qi and Mind-Intent is based on mutual dependence. But to actually employ Mind-Intent and the Qi within your Taijiquan practice can be very difficult, especially for beginning students. Yet, there really is no beginning method other than practicing the thirteen postures of the solo movements.

"What is absolutely necessary in the beginning, however, is to follow the imagination. For instance: when the two hands perform the *Pressing* gesture, there is an imagined intent to the front, as if an opponent were really there. At this time, within the palms of the hands there is no Qi which can be issued. The practitioner must then imagine the Qi rising up from the Dan-Tian into the spine, through the arms and into the wrists and palms. Thus, accordingly, the Qi is imagined to have penetrated outward onto the opponent's body.

"This use of imagination during initial study and practice will be difficult to trust and will not be susceptible to proof. Only after a long period of training will you be able to apply it in a natural manner, which is when the Qi penetrates the inner regions of the body. This occurs when [you actually experience sensations of] two circuits of the Qi within the gestures; then the Qi flows into the limbs of the body. When control of the Mind-Intent is achieved, the Qi will follow. At what point this occurs is immaterial as long as it is mobilized.

"In Taijiquan there are the fundamental principles of *'opening and closing,' 'fullness and emptiness,' 'inhaling and exhaling,'* and *'advancing and withdrawing.'* These are the training methods for circulating the Qi throughout the body. From these the body will become quite sensitive and alert, as will the muscles and tendons. The sense of touch will also become increasingly more acute. Thus, the spirit will be made active and alert."

Verses on Qi

"Within the text of *The Mental Elucidation of the Thirteen Kinetic Postures Treatise* there is a verse which states, 'If the Qi is not present, the Spirit of Vitality of the entire body and mind will be obstructed. When the Qi is present there is no need to exert muscular force, and without the Qi it is simply hardness.'

"In summary, the Qi will be useless unless it is dutifully regulated in an unconscious manner. Otherwise, the Qi will cause obstructions in your body, become unstable or fleeting, or abruptly produce a state of anger. At the time of having to issue the Qi, obstructive Qi, unstable Qi, and anger Qi will cause the feet to float and make the center of balance unsteady. This is what is meant to 'be without strength.'

"Taijiquan is said to center on the Qi of the Dan-Tian, [positive Qi]. This Qi is pure and tranquil. This tranquility makes it possible to be harmonious, this harmony makes it lucid, and lucidity makes the Qi safe and unobstructed. This prevents the Qi from producing scorching heat. In no way is this type of Qi similar to the above three negative kinds of Qi.

"The discussion of Qi within the text of *The Mental Elucidation of the Thirteen Kinetic Postures Treatise* is of great importance. For example:

'The mind moves the Qi so that it may sink deeply and penetrate the bones. When the Qi circulates freely and unhindered throughout the body, then it can easily follow the intentions of the mind.

'The Mind-Intent and Qi must interact in a lively manner to achieve both smoothness and circularity.

'The Qi is mobilized as though it were threading a pearl with nine crooked pathways; no hollow or corner is left unreached.

'The Qi should be nourished naturally so as not to have any injurious effects.

'Relax [Song] the abdomen, to allow the Qi to penetrate into the bones. Whether moving "to or fro" the Qi is to adhere to the spine.'

"Within *The Song of Thirteen Postures* it is said:
 'The Qi should be circulated throughout the body without the slightest obstruction.
 'When the Mind-Intent and Qi are the rulers, the bones and flesh follow their dictates.
 'When the Mind-Intent and Qi are regulated, it follows that the bones and flesh will become heavier.'

"These verses concerning the Qi are all of great importance. When learning these it is difficult to distinguish all of them from one another, especially when differentiating bright [positive] Qi from the scorching heat of the obstructive [negative] Qi.

"The relationship between the Mind-Intent and Qi is like that of an automobile; inside is the driver and an engine. The Mind-Intent is the driver and the Qi, the engine. Either of these would be seriously lacking without the other."

Chapter Three
Mobilizing the Qi

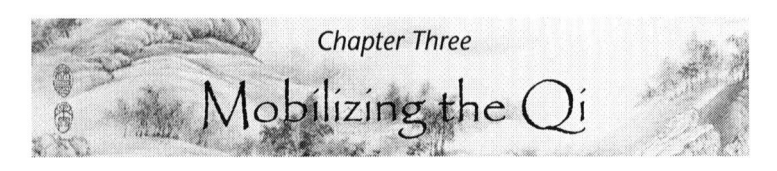

運氣

From understanding Mind-Intent and Qi, the Qi must be mobilized. This chapter explains the stages of Upper and Lower Level Breath, its relation to Before Heaven Qi and After Heaven Qi and how these two mutually mobilize each other. It further explains how the Heng Ha sounds work to stimulate Qi and to lay the foundation for tranquility. There is also a discussion of how these methods are applied in two-person drills.

"Taijiquan is praised by practicers as an internal style of boxing. They have three reasons for doing this. The first is because of the opinions of the scholarly community, which differentiates it from transcendentalism. The second reason involves its ingenious skills of *restraining, seizing, grasping,* and *closing* the actions of attackers. These counteroffensive movements are internal and formless. Third, one can employ the circulation of the internal Qi.

"Within the beginning procedures of Taijiquan breathing, inhalation and exhalation are done through the nose and not the mouth. Ordinarily one uses the nose to inhale and the mouth to exhale, but this is not done here. Also, when reaching a high level of skill, the Qi within the chest and stomach will become internally hot and you will be able to distinguish the stimulation of the *Upper* and *Lower Level Breath*. These are also called Before Heaven Qi [Before Heaven Breath] and After Heaven Qi [After Heaven Breath]."

The intrinsic energies of *restraining, seizing, grasping,* and *closing* are explained in my book *Tai Ji Jin—The Intrinsic Energies of Taijiquan*—a companion translation from Chen's book. Briefly, *Restraining* means to collapse the blood vessels of the opponent. *Seizing* means to obstruct the Qi meridians of the opponent. *Grasping* means to damage the tendons of the opponent. *Closing* means to close the vital Qi cavities of the opponent. These four energies are really the apex of Taijiquan self-defense and energy skills.

Upper Level Breath (上層氣, Shang Ceng Qi) represents the inhalation that is directed from the Dan-Tian upward along the spine to the Ni-Wan cavity on top of the head. *Lower Level Breath* (下層氣, Xia Ceng Qi) corresponds to the exhalation that is directed from the Ni-Wan down through the thorax into the Dan-Tian along the front of the body.

The terms Before Heaven Qi and After Heaven Qi are the proper Daoist names for Upper and Lower Level Breathing. Before Heaven Qi is associated with the inhalation, as it ascends to Heaven; After Heaven Qi is associated with the exhalation, as it descends to Earth.

Some books have suggested, erroneously, that Upper Level Qi and Lower Level Qi is a matter of directing the breath into the lungs and the abdomen respectively. This is, however, as the text later clarifies, both a "conflicting and unorthodox method."

"When exhaling the Upper Level Breath, you must exhale from the nose; then, immediately afterward the Lower Level Breath will return and descend into the Dan-Tian. When inhaling the Upper Level Breath, draw it in through the nose and then, immediately afterward, the Lower Level Breath will return to the Dan-Tian to be pressed again upward along the spine. These conditions are commonly called 'Circulating the Qi.'

"If you simply practice the orthodox art of Taijiquan, the correct levels can be attained and all the stages penetrated. Yet, in the beginning be sure to not become excessive about training. Avoid self-imposed obstacles to your martial art practice. Seek only to practice postures in a nonaggressive manner. Inhale and exhale naturally. The entire body should be open and relaxed, nothing more; otherwise the body might reject or oppress the proper maintenance of the Qi. Guide and compel the Qi to sink into the Dan-Tian.

"It is certainly easy to be influenced onto an unorthodox path that conflicts with this teaching. This can create problems in the lower extremities, such as bleeding piles, hernias, or other similar afflictions.

"After having attained a proper level of skill, the breath will produce Qi. But how to put it into use? If you do not pay attention to the principles, higher spiritual states will not be experienced.

"*The Mental Elucidation of the Thirteen Kinetic Postures Treatise* says, 'With proper breathing you can become alert and lively.' Mind-Intent is then breathing with movement. They should be as inextricable as the joint motion of two hands clapping together. For if you inhale, you must exhale; and if you exhale, you must inhale. The inhalation becomes insubstantial and the exhalation becomes substantial (as yin becomes yang and yang becomes yin).

"Afterward you will understand how the Qi naturally makes the body alert and lively; otherwise, the substantial and insubstantial will always be indiscernible. This is how to truly examine the errors made in practicing Taijiquan, because Taijiquan, in its most important aspect, is the understanding of substantial [yang] and insubstantial [yin].

"In general, these teachings were conferred only to family disciples. The teachings were divided into two sections, internal and external. The internal trains in the inhalation and exhalation of Qi. The external trains in the boxing techniques and gestures. Usually, just the essentials of the external methods were taught and the internal aspect was most often not transmitted. This withholding of information only disrupts and injures the proper principles of practice. It results in people being unable to comprehend naturalness and spontaneity. Possibly, in time, you could intuitively comprehend its secrets. But for those who do know, to not impart their knowledge only results in a continuing practice of not showing others.

"The original books acted as a teacher to the beginner, but everyone should also have a teacher. It is impossible to acquire the teachings solely through books. This would be like food caught in the throat which must be vomited up. You need a teacher to give detailed accounts of both the method and practical use.

"Generally, keep performing the circular movements of Taijiquan. When the hands *push out*, you exhale; when *withdrawing* the hands, inhale. *Rising*, you inhale; *sinking*, exhale. *Lifting*, you inhale; *lowering*, exhale. *Opening*, you inhale; *closing*, exhale. When moving the feet or turning the body in transition during a gesture, you perform a short breath.

"*Short Breath:* these are short inhalations and exhalations. You still inhale and exhale, but the mental image here is of a slight stopping or restraining.

"When performing Sensing-Hands: exhale on *Pushing;* exhale on *Pressing;* inhale on *Rolling-Back* and exhale on *Warding-Off.* When being the object of Rolling-Back, perform naturally a short breath [a quick inhalation when sensing the opponent's energy and then an exhalation when actually Rolling-Back]; seek also a quiet mind. With a tranquil mind you can see and listen to the actions of the opponent so as not to make a serious mistake.

"Being the object of Press or Push and unable to perform a repeated inhalation, change to an exhalation, because to employ another inhalation [to force it] advances the Qi, dispersing it into the four limbs. The opposite here is also true, concerning the exhalation. In either case learn not to force the breath—do not force an inhalation after having already inhaled; do not force an exhalation after having already exhaled. Naturally inhale and exhale according to circumstances.

"In regard to inhaling and exhaling within the Rolling-Back posture: when first sensing the opponent's attack, exhale; with *Shouldering*, exhale; with Pushing, exhale; Rolling-Back, inhale. When being the object of Shouldering, inhale. When the object of Rolling-Back, first do a short exhalation and then inhale; when turning the body back, seize the opportunity for Pushing and even though not yet Pushing, perform a short exhalation and inhalation when the opponent steps but has not yet issued the intrinsic energy. Also, when activating the short inhalation and exhalation, watch and listen with a tranquil mind to better acquire *Sticking* and *Adhering* intrinsic energy.

"The inhalations and exhalations for the Sword, Saber, Staff, and Dispersing-Hands, etc., along with their practical applications, are the same as with the circular form. When the hands [or weapon] are extended, you exhale; withdrawing the hands, you must inhale; rising, you inhale; descending, you exhale; opening, you inhale; closing, you exhale. Your perception or sensations are the guide here, but do not make repeated reference to them, for every situation is different."

Moving the Qi

"Regarding the methods for mobilizing the internal Qi, distinguish between the Before Heaven, which mobilizes the After Heaven, and the After Heaven, which mobilizes the Before Heaven. These are the two types of mobilization:

The actual instructions for these methods of Qi mobilization are given in the next chapter, "Taijiquan and Meditation."

Xian Tian and Hou Tian

— Ni-Wan

(Exhalation)

After Heaven Qi
Lower Level Breath

Also called:
Withdrawing the Yin
Yin Convergence
(Yin Fu)
The White Tiger

Dan-Tian

(Inhalation)

Before Heaven Qi
Upper Level Breath

Also called:
Advancing the Yang
Yang Fire
(Hou Yang)
The Green Dragon

1) The Before moves the After. It is said, *'The Before Heaven causes the After Heaven to move.'*

"The Qi in the Dan-Tian moves down and penetrates into the Sea Bottom (海底, Hai Di) cavity [coccyx area], then directly travels to the Tail Gate cavity [the tip of the tail bone] where it rises and connects with the spine to continue moving upward, threading through the Jade Pillow cavity [the occiput on back of the head], and to the Heavenly Spiritual cavity [top of the forehead] points.

"Moving downward it passes through the front of the forehead, through the center of the raphe of the upper lip, throat, and down into the stomach. Reaching the navel it returns to the origin [Dan-Tian].

2) The After moves the Before. It is said, *'The After Heaven mobilizes the Before Heaven.'*

"The Qi of the Dan-Tian moves upward. As it does it passes through the navel, abdomen [solar plexus], throat [Adam's apple], the raphe of the upper lip, and the front of the forehead. It continues through the Heavenly Spiritual cavity [forehead], and Jade Pillow cavity [occiput] points. It connects with the spine and moves down to the Tail Gate cavity [tailbone], then passes through the Sea Bottom cavity [coccyx], moves upward and returns to the origin [Dan-Tian].

"The above style [#2] is directly opposite to the first style. This type of Qi mobilization, especially to the beginner, is very difficult to prove. But eventually you can pass beyond this condition of doubt and realize the internal Qi. The above are the two types of circulation of the internal Qi.

"Upon completing the solo training of the exercises contained within this book you should apply this to external use and begin training the issuance of intrinsic energy with others [Sensing-Hands practice]. Then you will be able to correctly observe its use. If not, when needing to issue energy, you will be defeated or harmed and all your efforts will have been in vain.

"In martial arts, the Push is the highest level within Taijiquan. It is not enough to just circulate the Qi within yourself. As stated, it is experience with issuing energy that enables you to defeat an opponent. Because of the internal Qi, whether rising or descending, moving to or fro, you will be aware of the Qi gathering in the hands. This will reveal to you how truly subtle this form of kung fu really is. Without much basic training this will be difficult to apprehend."

Heng and Ha

"There are intrinsic sounds within the inhalation and exhalation called 'Heng Ha.' Following this profound skill enables you to unite these sounds with the breath and mouth, but to be precise it is the navel [Dan-Tian] which works the inhalation and exhalation."

> *Heng Ha* is commonly translated as "to hum and haw." It is also a reference to two fierce looking spirits usually guarding a temple gate or sometimes painted on the doors. Heng (pronounced "hun") is commonly associated with the sound we make when being frightened. Ha, to the sound associated with laughter.
>
> When practicing Taiji Qigong, Taijiquan solo forms, or two-person exercises, the sound of Heng Ha is kept inaudible. It creates a gentle and smooth vibration internally,

which benefits both the five viscera and the stimulation of Qi. It is important to direct the sound from the Dan-Tian, not the throat.

Heng Ha is a beginning stage of training the "Golden Bell Qigong," wherein the Qi protects the body against injury.

Intrinsic energy is what stimulates the Qi to be issued, otherwise the Qi may become stagnated. Heng Ha can likewise stimulate the intrinsic energy and Qi.

If the sound is projected from the Dan-Tian it can be tremendously powerful and frightening to an opponent. This is akin to a baby who can produce extremely loud shrieks from crying but never suffer a sore throat because the sound is produced from the Dan-Tian. Much like a good singer projects their voice from the lower abdomen.

"In both solo training and sparring with an opponent, the skill of Heng Ha is of great importance. Each one should be trained to the point of thoughtlessness, as though these words just emerge from the mouth. There are three principle reasons for training in Heng Ha:

"The first is to use these sounds so that the internal Qi will bring about comfort and tranquility. You can avoid being injured in an accident without having to use your martial arts skills.

"The second is to use these sounds so that the intrinsic energy of the entire body will stimulate the Qi to come out, without the slightest obstruction.

"The third is to use these sounds to frighten the opponent. His movements will then be disorganized; his spirit and mind confused. Whether you are advancing or withdrawing, he will misinterpret you, but you will exhibit self-control. Then you will be able to take advantage of his weakness and defeat him.

"These three secrets of Heng Ha have great use. Upon learning them you will eventually employ them without being aware of it."

"In the original manuscript within the *Taiji Quan Classic* called, 'Secret Songs' (歌訣, Ge Jue), it says: *'To abide by the Dan-Tian is to train the internal skill of Heng Ha. These two breaths are wonderful and inexhaustible. Activity is divided. In stillness it joins; in action it follows the curve and fully extends. Slowness and speed should be responded to accordingly. Following this principle you can thoroughly understand.'*

"Also, within the inner text of the old *Taiji Quan Treatise* it says: *'When dealing with another* [Sensing-Hands] *and moving "to and fro," sooner or later you must let loose and use Issuing Energy* (發勁, Fa Jin), *and this is as if shooting an arrow into the clouds. How much should one nourish the Qi? In one breath a loud sound, 'Ha' is made and then withdrawn immediately* [the more Qi the louder the sound]. *This is the oral transmission which was secretly handed down. Opening this gate one can see directly into the heavens.'*

"From [these excerpts] one can understand the profound uses of these two words Heng and Ha."

Methods of Qigong Breathing

In the Qigong and internal alchemy practices several breathing methods are incorporated. Before continuing further, it is best to introduce them here. It will be far easier to follow the instructions if each method of the breathing is explained first.

Cleansing Breath (清息, Qing Xi)

This method is applied before beginning any of the exercises or forms of Taijiquan. It aids in relaxing the body and breath, and rids the lungs of any impurities and tension. First, inhale through the nose deeply into the lower abdomen (expanding it) and then breathe out the mouth (contracting the lower abdomen). Repeat in succession nine times before practicing. This will help eliminate any congested air in the lungs, and help alleviate stress in the body.

Natural Breath (自息, Zi Xi)

There are two types of Natural Breathing, *Yin Natural Breath* (陰自息, Yin Zi Xi) and *Yang Natural Breath* (陽自息, Yang Zi Xi). The difference between them is that Yin Natural Breathing maintains a longer exhalation than inhalation, and Yang Natural Breathing maintains a longer inhalation than exhalation.

When inhaling, the abdomen expands, and it contracts during the exhalation. Each breath is inspired and expired through the nose with the tip of the tongue placed on the upper portion of the inside of the mouth. Natural Breathing is accomplished simply by putting all of your attention into the lower abdomen (Dan-Tian) so that there is no forcing of the breath to be deep and slow, rather it will be the Mind-Intent which regulates the breathing.

The first rule of Natural Breathing is just that, to be natural. Do not force the breath to be either long or deep. Let this happen naturally through practice. Use the Mind-Intent to keep the breath in the lower abdomen. Use the abdomen like a balloon or bellows to expand and contract it equally. Do not just push out the front of the stomach on inhalation and pull it inward on exhalation. Rather, on the inhalation you should sense an expansion of the breath on the lower spine, sides of the body, and front of the abdomen. On the exhalation, you should feel the contraction in a similar manner.

As you progress with Natural Breathing there will be a sense of the entire body breathing, feeling the inhalation expanding the very skin and muscles of the entire body, from the toes to the fingers, and contracting when exhaling. This is a very beneficial stage to reach as it will bring greater sensitivity and Qi to the body.

Embryonic Breathing (胎息, Tai Xi)

This breathing method is also called Reverse Breathing (反息, Fan Xi) and Immortal Breathing (仙息, Xian Xi). The abdomen contracts on the inhalation and expands on the exhalation, and each breath is inspired and expired through the nose with the tip of the tongue placed on the upper portion of the inside of the mouth. Reverse Breathing is accomplished by using the muscles of the lower abdomen—the inhalation (contraction of the abdomen) then pushes the Qi up along the spine, and the exhalation (expansion of the abdomen) pushes the Qi back down into the lower abdomen.

Embryonic Breathing is very useful for martial art concerns as the Qi can develop faster than with Natural Breathing. However, with Embryonic Breathing, tranquility is more difficult to achieve, because if practiced incorrectly or too forcefully it has the tendency to rapidly produce negative Qi, which can possibly create various psychological disorders. So, in practicing Embryonic Breathing with these exercises, it is best to do so when the body is ready and to do so in as relaxed a state as possible.

Embryonic Breathing is how we breathed inside the womb, and is why it is sometimes called Before Heaven Breath. When we leave the womb, we begin the After Heaven Breath. This type of breathing is crucial to internal alchemy, but is only used after feeling the effects of Natural Breathing. In brief, through use of the Yin Natural Breath a person will begin sensing tingling sensations in the body and wavelike motions in the body. These effects are signs of the body needing more yang energy, so Yang Natural Breathings should be performed. From Yang Natural Breathing there will be a greater sense of heat and vapor-like sensations in the body. It is at this point Embryonic Breathing should be employed to reverse the flow of Jing-Qi (the Elixir) up the spine.

Heng Ha Breathing (哼哈息, Heng Ha Xi)

This has two methods within these exercises, inaudible and audible. For inaudible you just internally sense and hear the drone of Heng Ha as you inhale and exhale. This is a very effective way to induce the Qi to mobilize in the body and the subtle meridians.

The audible use is primarily used for martial art purposes. When the Heng Ha method is mastered a person can let out a very primal sound, coming from the lower abdomen, that is completely alarming and disconcerting to an opponent.

In the exercise of Expressing the Qi (see p. 90), you internally sense and hear Heng as you inhale, but let out an audible Ha sound when exhaling. Attempt to let the sound come up from the Dan-Tian, not the throat. Doing so will greatly enhance your ability to express Qi out from your body.

Holding the Breath (閉氣, Bi Qi)
This breath is also called Tortoise Breathing (歸息, Gui Xi). In the exercises, primarily in the Taiji Qigong exercise, the more advanced practicers will hold the breath periodically at certain points in the form. This is done to attract and accumulate greater quantities of Qi. The very roots of Qigong stem from this idea of holding the breath to concentrate the Qi. The breath is always held after the inhalation and is maintained for either three or nine heartbeats, depending on the practicer's ability to do so. When holding the breath put all the attention in the cavity indicated and listen internally to the heart beats.

The One Breath (一氣, Yi Qi)
This is the apex of internal alchemy and Qigong methods—to breathe completely internally. Actually, there is no method for this, rather it is something that occurs unconsciously and spontaneously from continuous regulation of the breath. All the preliminary breathing methods are aids in which to experience this One Breath, or as Daoists refer to it, *True Breath* (真氣, Zhen Qi). The sensation of this breathing is unlike the normal breath, as you won't feel like you are breathing physically at all. Even if a feather were put beneath your nostrils it would not move, a mirror would not be fogged, nor will the body expand and contract even slightly.

Internally, however, you will sense a fuller breath than you could ever experience with normal breathing because it is the Qi and Mind-Intent that is controlling the breath and being generated from within the lower Dan-Tian (just as you did when in the womb), not the physical functions normally associated with breathing.

Chapter Four
Taiji Qigong

太極氣功

This chapter provides the directions for performing the 21-Posture Taiji Qigong Form. Externally this is a very easy exercise to learn. The difficult aspect of the exercise is the application of Mind-Intent and Qi so that you perform all the movements in conjunction with the breathing.

All the postures should be strung together smoothly and evenly. After learning all the postures and you are able to work the breath along with the movements, the advanced methods should then be applied. These advanced methods make use of breathing techniques like Reverse Breathing, Heng Ha Breathing, and Holding the Breath, as well as concentration upon certain Qi cavities (氣穴, Qi Xue) of the interior body to mobilize the Qi through them. Progress slowly, as rushing into the advance methods will do little good until your body and breath can function as one unit.

Procedures for Strengthening and Mobilizing Qi

"The vital importance of the Qi within a person's body was explained in the earlier sections, '*Mind-Intent and Qi*' and '*Mobilizing the Qi*.' However, the actual training procedures for these are not explained within the two earlier discourses. Here then is a simplified and elementary procedure for developing the Qi.

"The dissipation of Qi results in our death; consequently, we should fear losing it, as it is not easily accumulated. The ancient books on Qi attempted to explain these particulars in full detail, but they lacked the clarity needed.

"To perform the exercises for strengthening and mobilizing the Qi, the following principles must be applied:

"The breath must be in unison with the movements of the body, doing so with the rise and descent of either the Before Heaven Qi [inhale] or the After Heaven Qi [exhale], which are, respectively, related to Upper Level Breathing [directing the Qi and breath up the spine] and Lower Level Breathing [directing the Qi and breath down the front of the body]. Learning and practicing this enables you to directly follow in the footsteps of the ancient masters and to enter within the inner chambers of these methods.

"More than anything else, avoid being unwittingly sidetracked; otherwise, all your efforts will be in vain. These procedures for strengthening and mobilizing the Qi must be gradually trained and developed through regular practice if the internal Qi is to be stimulated and exhibited externally, as is the case with Taijiquan. When your environment does not permit you to practice Taijiquan—when there is no room in which to practice the circular movements and stepping actions—you should utilize this exercise.

"Taiji Qigong allows the muscles and bones to be stretched and expanded, causing the blood and Qi to unite, and increasing the internal energy of Qi. Half measures are not enough. You need to train diligently to accumulate Qi.

"In my observation of students and disciples from previous generations of the Yang family, many were well acquainted with this particular exercise of Taiji Qigong, but few had access to its secrets. The reason for this was that the family instructors were unwilling and unconcerned about teaching others [non-family members]. They trusted only themselves. How pitiful!

"Some people may be inclined to treat this exercise as just another form of Eight Brocades (八段錦, Ba Duan Jin) or deep breathing. Such exercises will, of course, produce some benefit, but far less than what can be achieved with Taiji Qigong. Strive to learn this method well; it should not be treated lightly."

Chen is referring here to a standing form of Eight Brocades. This standing form, along with various weapon sets was an attempt to emulate the Taijiquan system. In contradistinction, the original seated practice of Eight Brocades is a very ancient form of Dao Yin (導引, Daoist breathing exercises) attributed to Zhongli Quan (鐘離權, one of the Eight Immortals). Zhongli Quan was reportedly the teacher of Lu Dongbin (呂洞賓), another of the Eight Immortals and attributed founder of the *Complete Reality Sect* (全真派, Quan Zhen Pai) of Daoism. The seated exercises of Eight Brocades are extremely effective for replenishing the Three Treasures. In my opinion, as well as Chen's, however, the standing form of Eight Brocades is not as effective as the Taiji Qigong exercise explained in this book.

See my book *Qigong Teachings of a Taoist Immortal: The Eight Essential Exercises of Master Li Ching-Yun* for complete instructions on the seated practice of Eight Brocades, as well as the Eight Brocades Seated Qigong Exercises DVD.

"When performing deep breathing to produce Qi, you must seek to do it naturally. Whether inhaling or exhaling, it must be performed slowly and gradually. Each breath should be taken slowly and without restraint; it should not be repressed by being too regulatory, which produces negative circulation. It is expected that you will train carefully."

Taijiquan Qigong Exercise

The following pages describe and illustrate the twenty-one postures of the Taiji Qigong exercise. Always perform the Cleansing Breath method before beginning, doing so at least nine times. Learn the movements using Natural Breathing, both Yin Natural Breathing and Yang Natural Breathing. When feeling the sensation of heat in the body, then progress to Heng Ha Breathing. After experiencing the sensation of the Dan-Tian in the lower abdomen—feeling it as a solid or congealed object and a growing sense of heat in the body—then begin performing Embryonic Breathing. Holding the Breath should be practiced as well during the Embryonic Breathing stage of training, doing so at the end of each posture, as mentioned in my commentary notes. The notes also mention the specific Qi cavity to focus on while holding the breath.

Use Yin Natural Breathing (longer exhales) until you can go through the entire regime naturally. When heat begins to develop, or you have sensations of tingling or shaking movement in the lower abdomen and body, move on to Yang Natural Breathing (longer inhales). It is important to get through these two Natural Breathing stages before progressing to Heng Ha, Embryonic, and Holding the Breath methods, which maintain regulated breathing with inhales and exhales equal in length. The first stage of Taiji Qigong is to get the body and mind into a yin state so that Song energy can be achieved, thus ensuring the accumulation of Qi. The Qi cannot be mobilized if it is not first accumulated.

Do not be in a hurry to make progress, it is more important that the Dan-Tian is developed and sensed first so that the Qi can begin to accumulate there, then all the other breathing methods will be much more effective and beneficial. A quote from the *Zhuang Zi* (狀子) exemplifies this best, *"Slow up! Slow up! We're in a hurry."*

Original Illustrations of Taiji Qigong

The drawings and translations of the Chinese text within them are part of Chen Kung's original text and are included here for added reference. Chen Kung comments at the end of his work that some aspects of the drawings may be incorrect. In the case of the Taiji Qigong exercise, for example, the feet should be separated at shoulder-width distance, not together as shown, so that the Qi can flow freely through the coccyx region. Also, the circled Chinese text indicating inhales and exhales do not relate clearly to Chen Kung's instructional text, and, in some cases, his text is unclear, as each posture should begin with an inhale and conclude with an exhale. See notes with each posture.

In the text of the drawings the ideas of *Sink the Qi to the Dan-Tian* and *Adhere the Qi to the Spine* appear frequently. In the language of Taijiquan, they refer to performing the Lesser Heavenly Circuit. Therefore, when practicing the exercise, sense the inhalation of the breath on the back along the spine (Adhere the Qi to the Spine) and feel it descend on the front of the body (Sink the Qi to the Dan-Tian) when exhaling. In internal alchemy language these terms appear as Advancing the Yang Fire (陽火進, Yang Huo Jin) and Withdrawing the Yin Convergence (陰符退, Yin Fu Tui).

First Posture

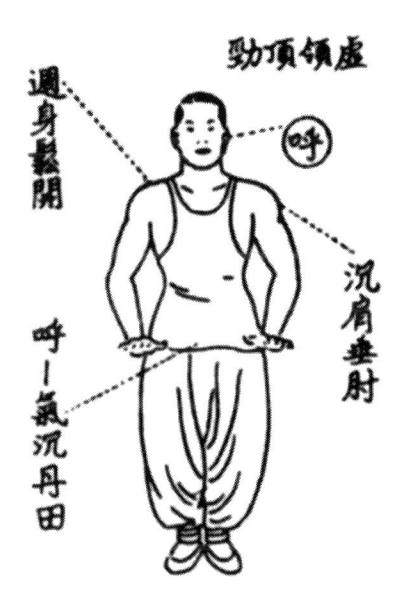

勁頂領虛
週身鬆開
呼
沉肩垂肘
呼―氣沉丹田

Gesture One
週身鬆開
The whole body should be relaxed and open.
虛領頂勁
Retain a light and sensitive energy on top of the head.
沉肩垂肘
Sink the shoulders and suspend the elbows.
呼― 氣沉丹田
Inhale　Sink the Qi to the Dan-Tian.
(Circle reads 吸 Xi "Inhale")

"Place both feet in line with one another in a fixed stance, with the head held erect. Retain a light and sensitive energy on top of the head. The eyes gaze levelly to the front. Place the tongue against the roof of the mouth and lightly close the lips and teeth.

This is the same stance as taken with the *Taijiquan Beginning Posture*. Exhale through the nose. The internal heat produced by the breath is divided into two levels, Upper and Lower.

"First, inhale through the nose and then, sinking the Qi gradually to the Dan-Tian, exhale. Lower the shoulders and elbows. Hollow the chest and raise the back. Press the palms of both hands downward; extend the fingertips to the front, but do not use muscular force. Slightly bend the arms and elbows. Relax the whole body. Raise the Spirit of Vitality; suspend the head from above as if by a string."

To begin learning this posture, you must first breathe through the nose so that the Qi can enter the hands. The Qi should be made to rise and descend, but follow a natural course.

This posture is one movement. The internal Qi is inhaled and exhaled to complete one circuit.

"Circuit" will throughout mean not only one complete cycle of inhalation and exhalation, but also a visualization of Qi ascending along the spine to the top of the head, and descending on the front of the body into the Dan-Tian.

Indications for holding the breath occur after the final exhale of each gesture. For Posture One, inhale and hold the Qi on top of the head in the Ni-Wan (Muddy Pellet) cavity, then exhale.

If necessary when first practicing holding the breath, you may inhale and exhale again before moving on to the following posture. This is called a "Restoration Breath" (還息, Huan Xi).

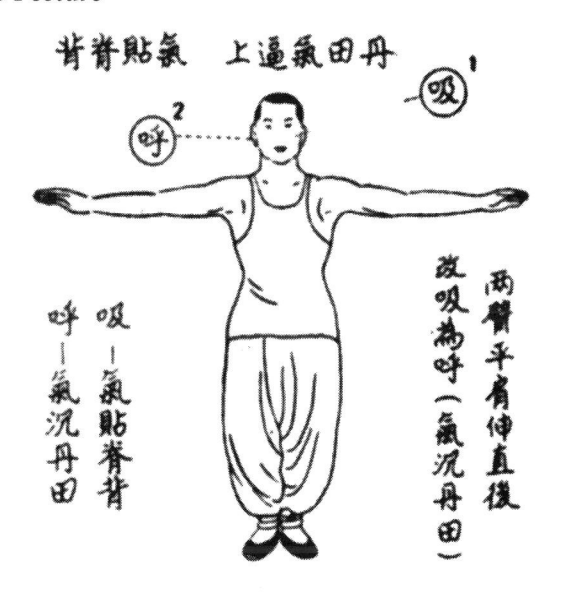

Second Posture

Gesture Two
上逼氣丹田
Press the Qi upward to the Dan-Tian.
氣貼脊背
Adhere the Qi to the spine.
兩臂平肩伸直後
The two arms are held out online with the shoulders
and extended straight back.
改吸為呼(氣沉丹田)
Change the inhalation to exhalation
(while sinking the Qi into the Dan-Tian).
吸　氣貼脊背
Inhale—Adhere the Qi to the spine.
呼—氣沉丹田
Exhale—Sink the Qi to the Dan-Tian.
(Circle 1 reads 吸 Xi "Inhale")
(Circle 2 reads 呼 Hu "Exhale")

"Both hands simultaneously move upward to the left and right sides. The arms stop upon reaching shoulder level. The palms face downward; the fingertips extend outward. The Qi gathers in, as the two hands open and separate and the inhalation enters through the nose. Direct the Qi from the Dan-Tian upward allowing it to adhere to the back of the spine. After the two hands are openly divided on line with one another, the movement momentarily stops. Alternate the inhalation to an exhalation. Sink the Lower Level Breath into the Dan-Tian."

Hold the Qi in the Double Pass cavity on the spine, middle of the back. Refer to the various graphics in Chapter Six and elsewhere in the book for locations of this and other Qi cavities.

In brief, for postures 1 and 21, hold the breath while sensing and visualizing the Qi in the Muddy Pellet (top of the head). For postures 6, 10, and 14, hold the Qi in the Jade Pillow (occiput) cavity, and for all other postures, hold the Qi in the Double Pass (middle of the back).

Third Posture

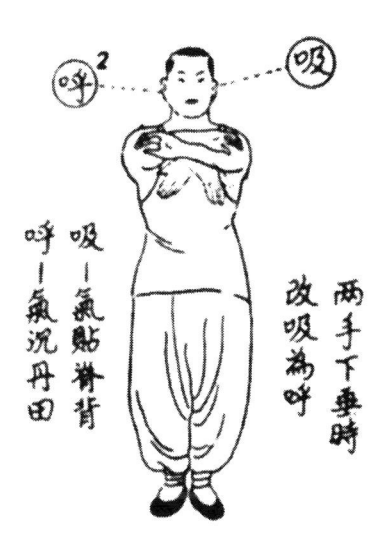

Gesture Three
兩手下垂時
When the two hands are hung downward,
改吸為呼
change the inhalation to exhalation.
吸—氣貼脊背
Inhale—Adhere the Qi to the spine.
呼—氣沉丹田
Exhale—Sink the Qi to the Dan-Tian.
(Circle 1 reads 吸 Xi "Inhale")
(Circle 2 reads 呼 Hu "Exhale")

"Both hands simultaneously move inward toward the front and then join. Inhale the Upper Level Breath through the nose and adhere the Qi to the spine. Then perform Lower Level Breathing and sink the Qi to the Dan-Tian.

"Place the right hand on top of the left, to form a crisscross shape with the palms facing down. Hollow the chest and raise the back. The two hands simultaneously turn downward with the palms facing toward the body. The fingertips hang downward. Inhale the Upper Level Breath; exhale the Lower Level Breath and sink the Qi to the Dan-Tian. This posture has two circuits of the Qi—two inhalations and two exhalations."

Hold the Qi in the Double Pass cavity on the spine, middle of the back.

Fourth Posture

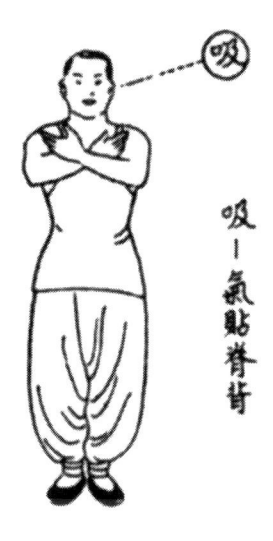

Gesture Four
吸 — 氣 貼 脊 背
Inhale—Adhere the Qi to the spine.
(Circle reads 吸 Xi "Inhale")

"Turn both hands inward and over in a circular manner, articulating the wrists so the left hand and wrist are inside the right hand and wrist. The left hand is inside between the body and the right hand. Both palms now face the body. After the hand movement, bend both knees so that the body lowers into a slight squatting position. Inhale, operating the Upper Level Qi, and adhering the Qi to the spine. This posture activates the internal Qi in one circuit."

Chen Kung doesn't mention exhaling in his instructions, but this posture, like all the others, ends with an exhale. He does say the posture activates the internal Qi in one circuit, which implies an inhale and exhale.

Hold the Qi in the Double Pass cavity on the spine, middle of the back.

Fifth Posture

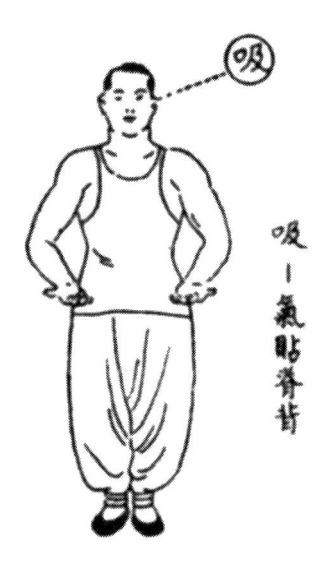

Gesture Five
吸 — 氣貼脊背
Inhale—Adhere the Qi to the spine.
(Circle reads 吸 Xi "Inhale")

"Both hands simultaneously turn upward and out then move downward and stop when they are beside the hips. Extend the fingertips to the front. During the hand movement raise the body upward by straightening your knees. Inhale the Upper Level Qi and adhere the Qi to the spine. Exhale the Lower Level Qi and sink the Qi to the Dan-Tian. There is no pause between Posture Four and Five so that the Qi makes one more circuit."

> Hold the Qi in the Double Pass cavity on the spine, middle of the back.

Sixth Posture

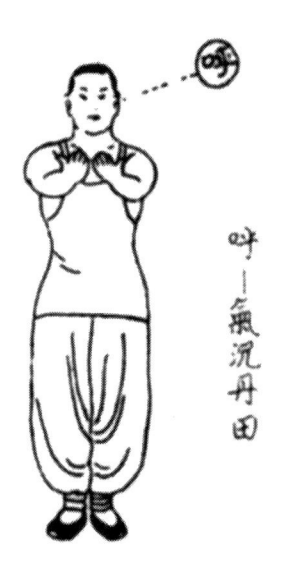

Gesture Six
呼— 氣 沉 丹 田
Exhale—Sink the Qi to the Dan-Tian
(Circle reads 呼 Hu "Exhale")

"With the palms still facing upward, move them forward, out and upward until both extend at the level of the chest. The palms face upward and the fingertips extend to the front. At the same time, bend both knees slowly, moving the body into a slight squatting position. Inhale, activating the Upper Level Qi and sink the Qi to the Dan-Tian. This posture has one circuit of the internal Qi."

Hold the Qi in the Jade Pillow cavity on back of the head.

Seventh Posture

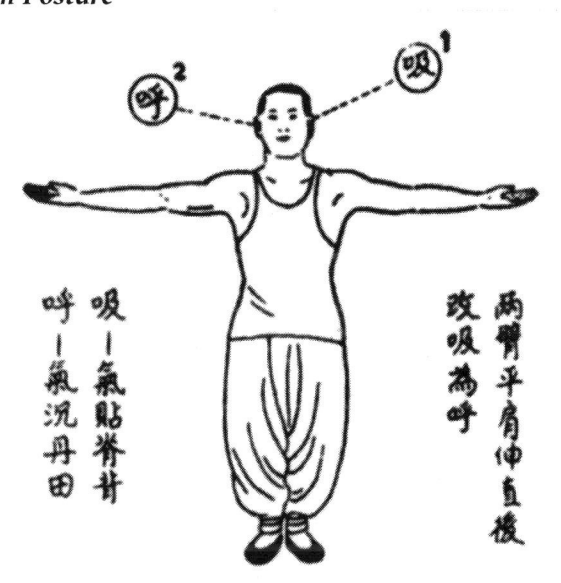

Gesture Seven
兩臂平肩伸直後
The two arms are held out online with the shoulders and extended straight back.
改吸為呼
Change the inhalation to exhalation.
吸—氣貼脊背
Inhale—Adhere the Qi to the spine.
呼—氣沉丹田
Exhale—Sink the Qi to the Dan-Tian.
(Circle 1 reads 吸 Xi "Inhale")
(Circle 2 reads 呼 Hu "Exhale")

"Separate both hands and move them to the left and right sides so that they are in line with the shoulders. The palms face upward and the fingertips stretch outward. As both hands open and separate, inhale to work the Qi, adhering it to the spine.

"After the hands open and separate, halt the movement momentarily. At this point exhale and gradually raise the body upward by slowly straightening the knees. During the exhalation sink the Qi to the Dan-Tian. This posture is one movement and completes one circuit of the internal Qi."

Hold the Qi in the Double Pass cavity on the spine, middle of the back.

Eighth Posture

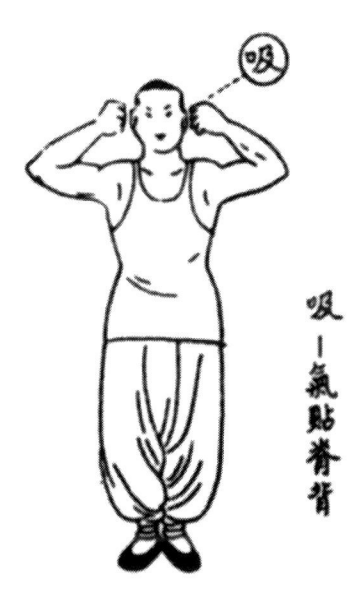

Gesture Eight
吸 — 氣 貼 脊 背
Inhale—Adhere the Qi to the spine.
(Circle reads 吸 Xi "Inhale")

"Turn both hands upward and inward, gradually forming them into fists as you do so. During this motion, move the fists until they reach the sides of the ears, with the 'tiger mouths' facing upward. Do not clench the fists too tightly. Very little energy should be used when raising the arms [no tension]. Relax and open the whole body; hollow the chest and raise the back. [During the exhale] bend the legs and lower the body into a squatting position. Inhale to activate the Upper Level Breath and adhere the Qi along the spine. Exhale to activate the Lower

Level Breath and sink the Qi to the Dan-Tian. This posture has one circuit of the internal Qi."

Hold the Qi in the Double Pass cavity on the spine, middle of the back.

Ninth Posture

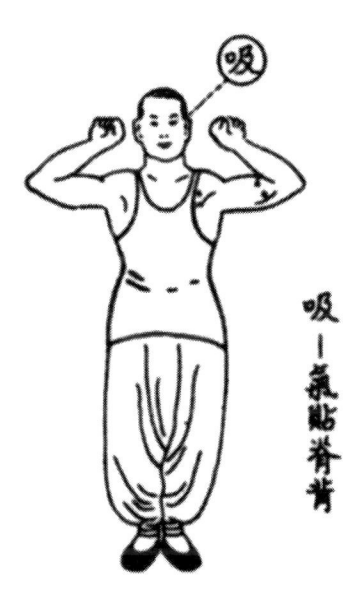

Gesture Nine
吸 — 氣 貼 脊 背
Inhale—Adhere the Qi to the spine.
(Circle reads 吸 Xi "Inhale")

"Both hands simultaneously turn over and out, so that the 'tiger mouths' face one another with the palms of the hands [in fist position] facing outward. Inhale to activate the Upper Level Breath and exhale to sink the Qi to the Dan-Tian. Along with the Eighth Posture, the internal Qi is strung together in one action, therefore, there is no pause in the movement. This posture has one circuit of the internal Qi."

>Hold the Qi in the Double Pass cavity on the spine, middle of the back.

Tenth Posture

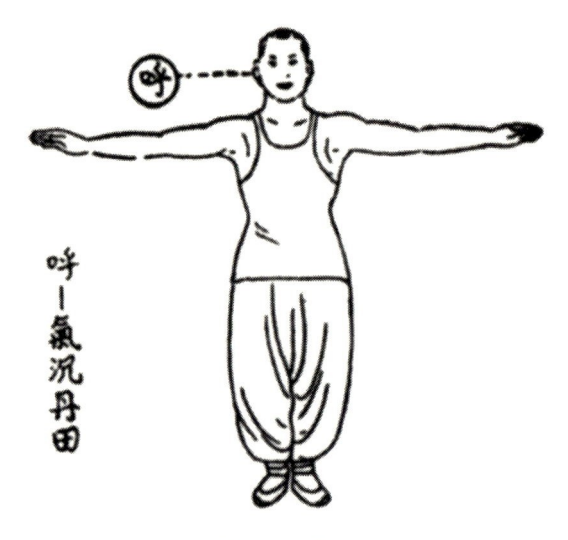

Gesture Ten
呼－氣沉丹田
Exhale—Sink the Qi to the Dan-Tian.
(Circle reads 呼 Hu "Exhale")

"Both fists change into open palms, while simultaneously moving to the left and right sides as the arms extend. The forearms move downward as the hands are opening. By the time the forearms are level with the shoulders [left arm off the left shoulder and right arm off the right shoulder] the palms face downward. The fingers stretch outward. Straighten the knees to slowly raise the body. Inhale to activate the Upper Level Breath and cause the Qi to rise upward along the spine. Exhale to sink the Qi to the Dan-Tian. This posture has one circuit of the internal Qi."

Hold the Qi in the Jade Pillow cavity on back of the head.

Eleventh Posture

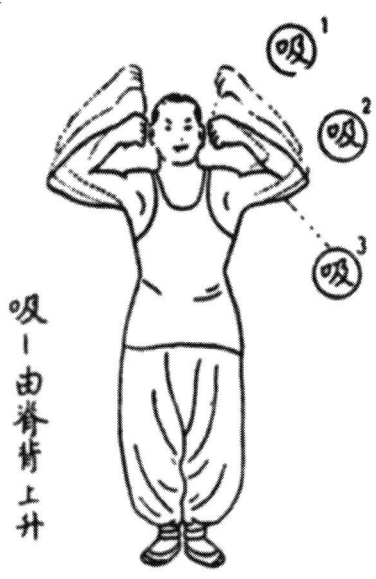

Gesture Eleven
吸 — 由脊背上升
Draw the inhale up the spine.
(Circle 1 reads 吸 Xi "Inhale"
(Circle 2 reads 吸 Xi "Inhale"
(Circle 3 reads 吸 Xi "Inhale"

"Move the hands inward and upward, by the ears with the 'tiger mouths' facing upward. Hollow the chest and raise the back. The knees bend to lower the body into a slight squatting position. This is just like the Eighth Posture. Inhale to activate the Upper Level Breath; exhale to activate the Lower Level Breath and sink the Qi to the Dan-Tian.

"Both fists simultaneously rise until they are beside the temples. The knees slowly straighten to raise the body gradually upward. Inhale to activate the Upper Level Breath, adhering the Qi to the spine."

"The two fists continue to rise upward until they are above the head. Exhale to activate the Lower Level Breath and sink the Qi to the Dan-Tian."

Chen Kung's commentary indicates two circuits of the Qi, but the circles suggest three. In this case, follow his instructions by inhaling and exhaling to draw the hands in below the ears. Then inhale while raising the hands to temple height, and exhale to raise them above the head, completing two circuits of Qi.

Hold the Qi in the Double Pass cavity on the spine, middle of the back.

Twelfth Posture

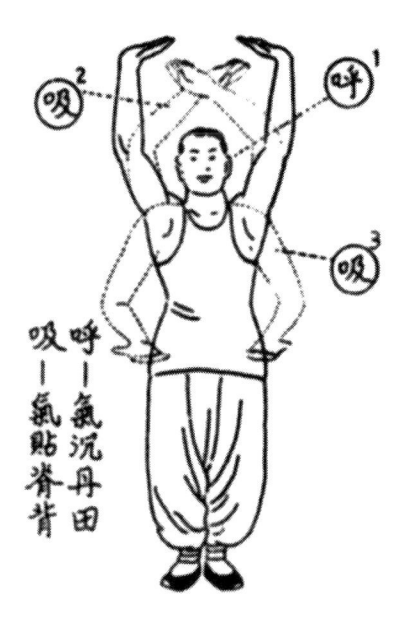

Gesture Twelve
呼 — 氣沉丹田
Exhale—Sink the Qi to the Dan-Tian.
吸 — 氣貼脊背
Inhale—Adhere the Qi to the spine.
(Circle 1 reads 呼 Hu "Exhale")
(Circle 2 reads 吸 Xi "Inhale")
(Circle 3 reads 吸 Xi "Inhale")

"Push both hands simultaneously upward as though to support something weighted, with the palms facing upward and the fingers of each hand pointing to those of the other. Raise the body slightly upward by straightening the knees and raising the heels off the ground. Inhale to activate the Upper Level Breath.

"Turn both hands inward so that they cross at the wrists. This cross-like position has the right hand on top and the left underneath with each palm facing outwards. Exhale the Lower Level Breath.

"Lower both hands simultaneously until they are beside the pelvic area, with the palms facing upward and the fingers pointing to the front. Lower the heels gradually."

"The original position is now restored, as in the Fifth Posture. Inhale to activate the Upper Level Breath and exhale to sink the Qi to the Dan-Tian. This posture has three movements and [three] circuits of the internal Qi."

Circuit 1: Inhale when pushing the hands upward; exhale to cross them. Circuit 2: Inhale and exhale while lowering the hands as they remain crossed in front of the chest. Circuit 3: inhale and exhale to continue the downward movement of the hands until they are beside the pelvic area, as in Posture 5.

Hold the Qi in the Double Pass cavity on the spine, middle of the back.

Thirteenth Posture

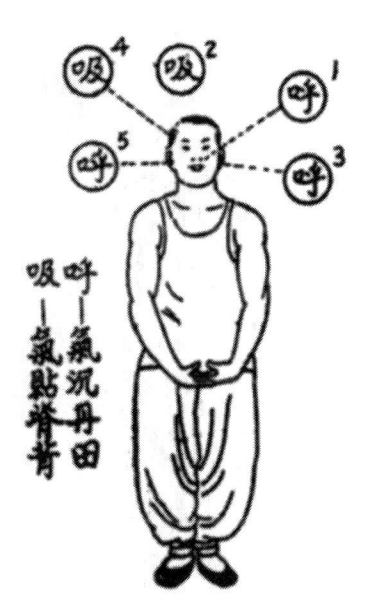

Gesture Thirteen

呼 — 氣沉丹田
Exhale—Sink the Qi to the Dan-Tian.
吸 — 氣貼脊背
Inhale—Adhere the Qi to the spine.
(Circle 1 reads 呼 Hu "Exhale")
(Circle 2 reads 吸 Xi "Inhale")
(Circle 3 reads 呼 Hu "Exhale")
(Circle 4 reads 吸 Xi "Inhale")
(Circle 5 reads 呼 Hu "Exhale")

"Hold the head erect. Turn both hands simultaneously inward so that they join in front of the lower abdomen. The palms face upward and the thumbs of each hand face one another. The left hand is above the right. Inhale so that the Qi adheres to the back, along the spine, and exhale to sink the Qi to the Dan-Tian.

"Both hands remain where they are. The head follows the waist and the torso in a leftward rotating posture. The gaze remains level as the head turns toward the back. Pause when the neck is unable to turn any further. Inhale to activate the Upper Level Breath and exhale to activate the Lower Level Breath.

"The head and waist return to the original position facing the front. Inhale and exhale to activate the Upper and Lower Level Breaths respectively.

"The head follows the waist by making a rightward rotating gesture. As the head turns, the gaze remains level. The head stops when it is unable to turn any further. The breath pattern is the same as described above.

"The head and waist return to the original position facing the front. Repeat the same breath pattern as above."

This posture has five circuits of the internal Qi.

> The instructions call for turning the head (by rotating the waist and body) to the left and right sides with a level gaze. You can augment these movements with two or three more rotations; however, this is optional. When turning, keep the head upright and straight, especially when pausing at the completion of a turn.
>
> Hold the Qi in the Double Pass cavity on the spine, middle of the back.

Fourteenth Posture

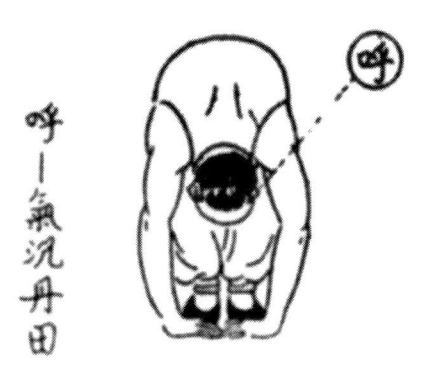

Gesture Fourteen
呼 — 氣 沉 丹 田
Exhale—Sink the Qi to the Dan-Tian.
(Circle reads 呼 Hu "Exhale")

"Turn both palms inward, over, and down so that the back of the hands face upward. Bend the upper part of the body over to the front into a low, stooping position. Place both palms upon the ground and hold the fingers of each hand opposite one another.

"The knees remain straight but not locked throughout the movement. When first practicing this posture, in case the hands are unable to be placed upon the ground, it will be quite adequate to stop and rest at a comfortable point, as this pressing gesture must not be forced. In time the waist will become more pliable and you will be able to naturally touch the ground. Exhale as you bend over to activate the Lower Level Breath and sink the Qi to the Dan-Tian.

"The movements of this posture circuit the Qi once. This posture must flow immediately after Posture Thirteen so that the exhalation can be maintained for both."

Although the text implies that no inhalation takes place for this posture, the idea is that the breathing is continuous and postures 13 and 14 should flow into each other without a pause. The inhalation then takes place before bending over and exhaling. As stated, each posture begins with an inhale and ends with an exhale, even when the drawings and Chen Kung's text indicate otherwise.

The movements of this posture can be augmented with either two or three more bending over and rising actions. Each addition will include another circuit of Qi, meaning you inhale when rising and exhale when bending back down.

Hold the Qi in the Jade Pillow cavity on the back of the head.

Fifteenth Posture

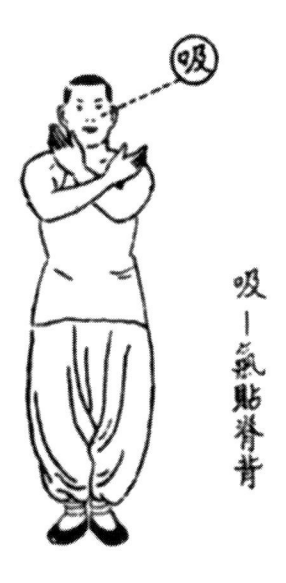

Gesture Fifteen
吸 — 氣 貼 脊 背
Inhale—Adhere the Qi to the spine.
(Circle reads 吸 Xi "Inhale")

"Raise the upper body to an upright position. Cross both hands so that the palms face inward. The right hand is on the outside and the left on the inside. Hollow the chest and raise the back. Now move the body down into a slight squatting position by gradually bending the knees. Inhale as you raise your upper body to an erect position, and exhale during the squatting motion."

Hold the Qi in the Double Pass cavity on the spine, middle of the back.

Sixteenth Posture

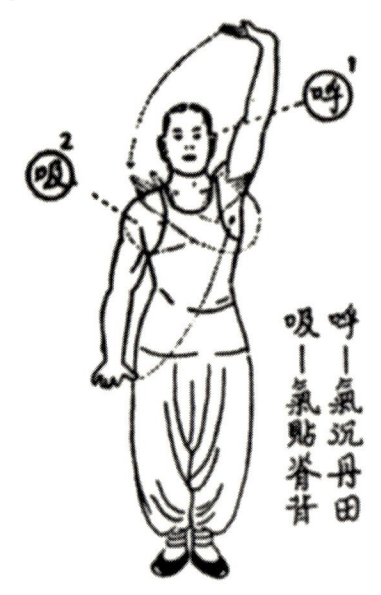

Gesture Sixteen
呼—氣沉丹田
Exhale—Sink the Qi to the Dan-Tian.
吸—氣貼脊背
Inhale—Adhere the Qi to the spine.
(Circle 1 reads 呼 Hu "Exhale")
(Circle 2 reads 吸 Xi "Inhale")

"Move the left hand upward as if you were lifting something with the palm. Simultaneously, press the right hand downward. The right palm faces down and the fingers extend to the front. Raise the body gradually upward as your knees straighten. The Upper Level Breath is stimulated when inhaling; exhaling enables the Qi to sink to the Dan-Tian.

"Move the left hand downward and the right hand upward at the same time and join them in the crisscross position in front of the chest. Now the left hand is on the outside and the right hand on the inside. Hollow the chest and raise the back as your body slowly sinks into a squatting position with both knees bending. Inhale to activate the Upper Level Breath and adhere the Qi to the spine. Exhale to sink the Qi to the Dan-Tian."

Hold the Qi in the Double Pass cavity on the spine, middle of the back.

Seventeenth Posture

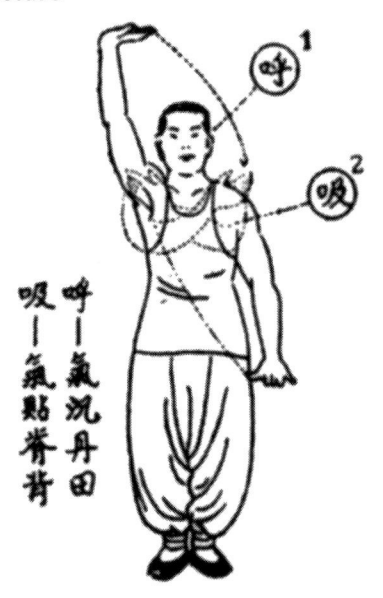

Gesture Seventeen
呼 — 氣沉丹田
Exhale—Sink the Qi to the Dan-Tian
吸 — 氣貼脊背
Inhale—Adhere the Qi to the spine.
(Circle 1 reads 呼 Hu "Exhale")
(Circle 2 reads 吸 Xi "Inhale")

"Move the right hand upward as if you were lifting something with the palm facing upward. Press the left palm down at the same time and extend the fingers to the front. Raise the body gradually upward as your knees slowly straighten. Inhale to activate the Upper Level Breath and adhere the Qi to the spine. Exhale to sink the Qi to the Dan-Tian.

"Move both hands to the front of the chest and join them in a crisscross position. This is just like the Fifteenth Posture. Hollow the chest and raise the back. The body slowly sinks into a slight squatting position as you bend both knees. Inhale to activate the Upper Level Breath and adhere the Qi to the spine; exhale to activate the Lower Level Breath and sink the Qi to the Dan-Tian."

Hold the Qi in the Double Pass cavity on the spine, middle of the back.

Eighteenth Posture

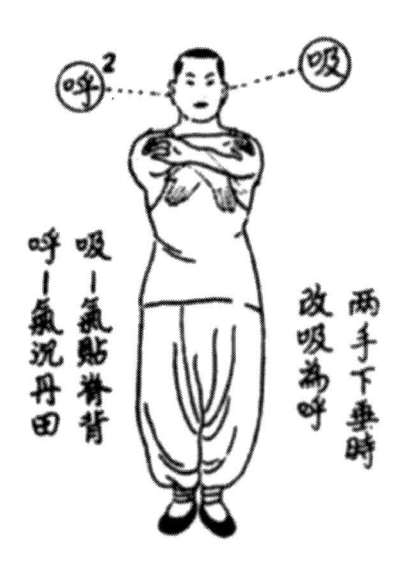

Gesture Eighteen
兩 手 下 垂 時
When the two hands are hung downward,
改 吸 為 呼
change the inhalation to exhalation.
吸 — 氣 貼 脊 背
Inhale—Adhere the Qi to the spine.
呼 — 氣 沉 丹 田
Exhale—Sink the Qi to the Dan-Tian.
(Circle 1 reads 吸 Xi "Inhale")
(Circle 2 reads 呼 Hu "Exhale")

"Turn both hands so that the palms face inward and the fingers hang downward. Raise the body by straightening the knees.

Inhale to activate the Upper Level Breath and exhale to sink the Qi to the Dan-Tian."

Hold the Qi in the Double Pass cavity on the spine, middle of the back.

Nineteenth Posture

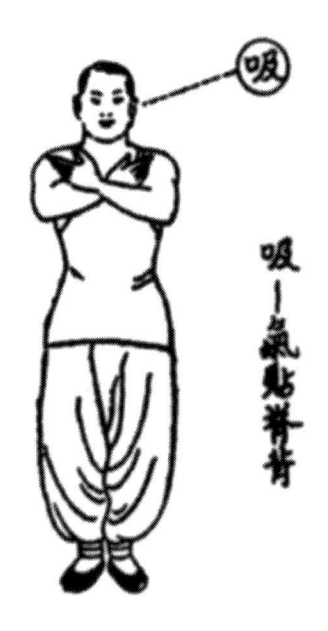

Gesture Nineteen
吸 — 氣貼脊背
Inhale—Adhere the Qi to the spine.
(Circle reads 吸 Xi "Inhale")

"Turn both hands so that they circle inward, upward, and over. The right hand turns until it is closest to the body. Both palms now face inward. The knees bend to lower the body into a squatting position. Inhale to adhere the Qi to the spine and exhale to sink the Qi to the Dan-Tian."

Hold the Qi in the Double Pass cavity on the spine, middle of the back.

Twentieth Posture

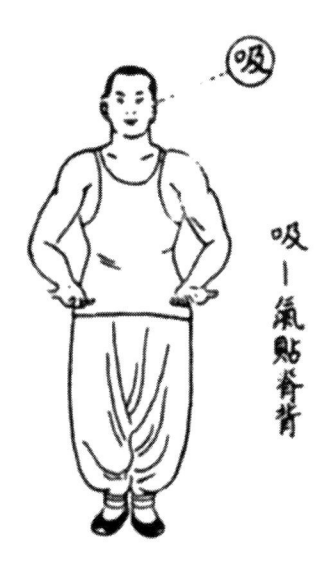

Gesture Twenty
吸 — 氣 貼 脊 背
Inhale—Adhere the Qi to the spine.
(Circle reads 吸 Xi "Inhale")

"Move both hands downward toward the rear and position them beside the pelvic area. The palms face upward and the fingers extend to the front. Gradually raise the body upward, by straightening the knees slightly. Inhale to activate the Upper Level Breath and exhale to sink the Qi to the Dan-Tian.

"This posture has both an inhalation and an exhalation, with one circuit of the internal Qi. It involves the same movement as Posture Five; therefore, there is no pause between this and the previous posture."

Hold the Qi in the Double Pass cavity on the spine, middle of the back.

Twenty-First Posture

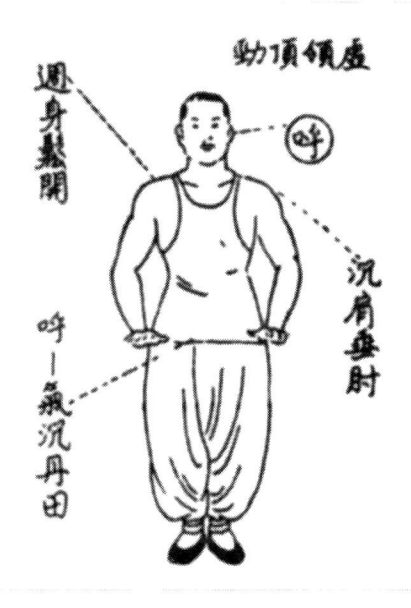

Gesture Twenty-One
週身鬆開
The whole body should be relaxed and open.
虛領頂勁
Retain a light and sensitive energy on top of the head.
沉肩垂肘
Sink the shoulders and suspend the elbows.
呼—氣沉丹田
Inhale—Sink the Qi to the Dan-Tian.
(Circle reads 呼 Hu "Inhale")

"Raise both hands upward to the left and right sides respectively until they are beside the rib area. Turn the palms down and lower them while your body rises as the knees straighten. This returns you to the original position of First Posture.

"This posture flows directly after the last one, so that the exhalation is maintained from one to the other. When exhaling, sink the Qi to the Dan-Tian.

"After completing the entire set of these gestures, stop and rest for a short period; then walk about to circulate the Qi and blood. Return to the original position and rest."

The text in the drawing says, "Inhale," which is incorrect because it is connected with "Sink the Qi to the Dan-Tian," which is done with an exhale, as Chen Kung and the other drawings say everywhere else. Like Posture 14, Chen Kung doesn't mention the inhale, but it takes place as you raise the arms. Exhale as you turn the palms over and lower the hands to the starting position.

Hold the Qi on top of the head in the Ni-Wan cavity.

Chapter Five
Qigong Stances

氣 功 步

The first of the supplementary Qigong exercises is called Expressing the Qi—a type of shaking motion that is to be felt more internally, feeling the energy from the Dan-Tian up the spine into the arms and out the fingertips. This will help balance the energy in your body, for too many Taijiquan practicers concentrate only on the accumulation of Qi, not on the expression of it.

The second exercise, Ma Pu (馬步, Riding a Horse Stance), is primarily a breathing exercise and secondarily a standing meditation. Again, treat this exercise as you would Taiji Qigong. All the same principles apply. Also, be patient, starting with a few minutes each day. Progress cautiously and with discretion.

The third exercise, Chuan Zi (川字),[1] is in essence a standing meditation. The key to these exercises is not in making the legs strong (in a muscular sense), but to apply Song (relaxation). When feeling the legs tense, mentally let the tension go. After a long, continued period of letting go, the legs will become softer and more relaxed, as real strength comes from Song, not from exertion of muscles.

> 1. This term doesn't translate well into English because the meaning is that the body should be in a position similar to the character 川 (Chuan).

The fourth exercise, Cai Tui (採腿), literally means "Pulling Leg." The importance of this exercise lies in unifying the body to express the Jin and Qi in the limbs simultaneously. Again, it is relatively easy to perform, but difficult to master internally.

These four exercises should be practiced daily, but first study the text thoroughly so you have a good understanding of not only their purpose, but the functions as well. Do not be anxious. Take your time exercising them a little each day, building up gradually to make more repetitions.

Expressing the Qi
"After practicing the entire set of Taiji Qigong exercises (or the Taijiquan solo form) perform these Qigong stances."

Preparation
"Separate both feet so that they are parallel to each other with the distance being slightly broader than the width of the shoulders. Drop the body into a horse stance, a low squatting position with the knees well bent."

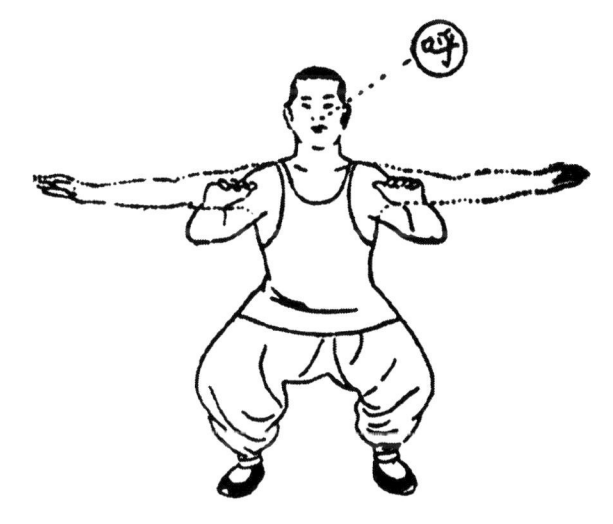

"The upper body must be upright and erect. Retain a light and sensitive energy on top of the head. Relax the waist and buttocks. Hollow the chest and raise the back. Sink the shoulders and lower the elbows. Draw in the buttocks. Bend both arms with the fingers pointing forward and the palms facing downward."

Movement
"Keeping the hands, arms and knees in place, use the energy of your waist and legs and at your discretion perform a shaking motion [expressed out the fingers and hands of both arms] one hundred or two hundred times.

"After completing these shaking motions, separate both arms levelly to the left and right sides with the fingers stretched outward and the palms facing downward. Again perform the same shaking motions one hundred or two hundred times.

"Lastly, rotate the body (to the left side and then the right side) to circulate the blood and Qi. This will put the body and mind in good spirits. What could be more advantageous than this? Consequently, this exercise is really indescribable!"

> The idea here is to internally create a vibration, originating in the Dan-Tian and coming through the shoulders and spine and then out the fingers. This vibration is not to be violent or forced, it is more akin to the idea of lashing out a whip, where the length of the whip (analogous to the length of the arms) is sent outward and snapped at the tip (analogous to the hands and fingers). The whole body should be relaxed. Inhale and rise up slightly, then sink and exhale—at the point of exhaling visual the Qi coming from the Dan-Tian, up the spine, and out the arms and hands. Thus creating a whip-like action of the arms and hands. This practice is also similar to that of Taiji Sword, wherein the blade of the sword is caused to vibrate by using the whole body as one unit.
>
> In this exercise also make use of the Heng Ha sounds with a short inhalation and longer exhalation, but do so inaudibly.

The purpose of this exercise is twofold:
1. In the Taiji Qigong exercise you are stimulating and accumulating Qi. This exercise then harmonizes the body by releasing it so that "scorching Qi" is not developed.
2. A foundation for learning to issue Qi off the spine and out the fingertips. Later, as you develop intrinsic energy, this will enhance your ability for Fa Jin (Issuing Energy).

Post Stances

"The Post Stances (椿步, Zhuang Bu) of Taijiquan are divided into two types: Ma Bu and Chuan Zi. Generations in the past who practiced the Taijiquan forms first practiced these two types of stances. This would make it possible for the intrinsic energy to also develop in the lower extremities [feet and legs], so to prevent drifting and floating."

> Regarding *Post Stances,* Zhuang Bu has two primary meanings: to stand like a post, or stake, and a buoy. The idea being expressed is that of being upright, rooted, and maintaining central equilibrium.

"The present generation seems to prefer to training within the confines of Sensing-Hands. For this reason, there are these methods of stance training, which are similar to that of building a foundation for a house. The foundation must be strong; otherwise, it could not support the topmost chambers in a high tower or the high ceilings of a large mansion. How could a weak foundation support anything above it?

"Unfortunately, few students take this work to hand. To progress gradually, begin practicing the circular forms of the Taijiquan postures and the exercises of Sensing-Hands; but take note, inexperience in [training] these stances has the consequence of there being no skill in the legs and feet and your center of balance can easily be tilted.

"Earlier writings on this subject urged that these stances be learned and that great attention be paid to them. If these stances are foregone then when performing the circular forms, the legs will not be seated firmly and you will not find precision in the posture movements. Likewise, when performing Sensing-Hands, with one easy pull that person will be bent over; with one push his center of balance will be disrupted and he will be thrown back. Consequently, if you wish to train in true kung-fu and do not practice Post Stances, you will be unsuccessful; these must be practiced! It is unimportant whether the period of practice is long or short, the important thing is to establish consistency. Simply do them on a regular basis. Even after one month they will prove their effectiveness. The following is a breakdown of the training procedures."

Riding a Horse Stance
"Maintain the center of balance between the legs, with the torso upright and straight. Suspend the head and relax the waist. Hollow the chest and raise the back. Sink the shoulders and hang the elbows. The Wei Lu [tail-bone area] is centered and upright. The eyes gaze intently at the hands. Gather the Qi and concentrate the spirit. Inhale and exhale through the nose. Bend and curve the two arms, with both hands out front and the palms directly facing one another as if holding a ball."

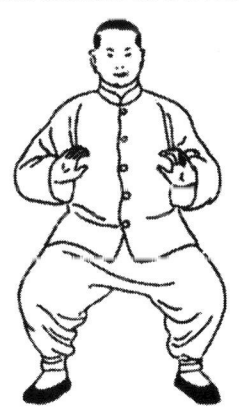

"Now distinguish between doing an ascent and descent with the body. The ascent: the body rises slightly upward and the two hands open slightly. Work the Qi on the inhalation and adhere it to the spine. On the descent the body moves slightly downward into a seated position and the hands close slightly. Work the Qi on the exhalation and sink it into the Dan-Tian.

"*Brief summary:* The two hands open and close once during each complete breath. They operate on a similar basis to the motion of the lungs when one is breathing.

"Beginners should pause five minutes in this position [after rising and sinking numerous times]. Gradually pause for a longer and longer span of time [possibly thirty minutes or so].

"Afterward, through time, the lower extremities [waist, legs, and feet] will acquire the skill of rootedness and the four limbs and entire body will have intrinsic energy. Externally everything will be substantially augmented and internally the Dan-Tian will be well nourished."

Chuan Zi Stances

"Stand erect. Step out with the right foot one-half step to the front and place the heel on the ground with the toes raised slightly upward. Bend the left leg. Separate the two feet so they are about one foot apart. The upper body is upright and the buttocks do not protrude. Hollow the chest and raise the back. Retain a light and nimble energy on top of the head. Center the Wei Lu (尾廬,

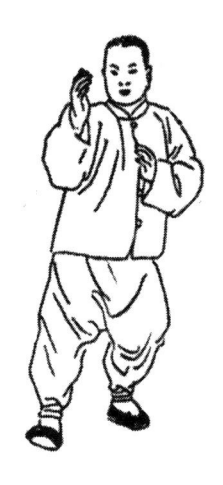

literally the 'Tail Bone') so that it is upright. Do not wander in thought or be anxious."

"With each inhalation adhere the Qi to the spine. With each exhalation sink the Qi into the Dan-Tian.

"Move the body down into a low squatting position, with the greater part of the body's weight on the left leg. Bend the two arms slightly and extend both hands forward. Sink the shoulders and hang the elbows. Straighten the wrists; bend the fingers slightly. They should be divided and open [relaxed]. The right hand is in front and the left hand is behind, being somewhat close to the front of the chest. The palms face one another, but are not parallel.

"The upper body consists of shoulders, elbows, and wrists. The lower body consists of hips, knees, and feet. Each of them are related—shoulders and hips, elbows and knees, wrists and feet.

"The entire body should be light and nimble, without a trace of external muscular exertion. It is essential to seek naturalness.

"This style is *Lifting Hands* within the Taijiquan Thirteen Postures, and it is exactly the same as Chuan Zi. The [instructions describe] the right style. The left style of Chuan Zi is similar to the right style; the difference being that the left hand and left foot are extended out to the front. The appearance of the left style is just like that of the posture, *Hands Playing The Guitar*, which is contained within the Taiji Thirteen Postures.

"When practicing the forms of post stances, whether for long or short periods, be consistent in your practice. Both the Mind-Intent and Qi are internal. Within one's body, especially the waist and legs, is the kung-fu of intrinsic energy. Each of these—Mind-Intent, Qi, and intrinsic energy—have limitless benefit.

"Within the Pushing Posture of Taijiquan there is *Advancing, Withdrawing, Looking-Left, Gazing-Right,* and *Central-Equilibrium.* They are also contained within the Post Stances, and the weapon styles. These, *'Five Attitudes,'* are very important within any of the Taijiquan practices.

"Previous generations trained in these kung-fu stances every day without fail for ten years or more. They did this to develop these postures and attain the results of the cultivation of Mind-Intent, Spirit, and Qi. Therefore, if taking up the practice of Taijiquan do so without negligence. In regard to all the other solo postures in the Taijiquan Thirteen Postures, any one of them will do for practicing Post Stances. Ideally, practice each one as a Post Stance."

> *Thirteen Postures* (十三勢, Shi San Shi). Normally *shi* is translated as "postures," but should be considered more as power, strength, and influential activity. These Thirteen Postures are the primary functions of Taijiquan. In earlier Taijiquan history, the form was originally called "Taijiquan Thirteen Postures." The names of the postures are:
>
> 1) Warding-Off
> 2) Rolling-Back
> 3) Pressing
> 4) Pushing
> 5) Pulling
> 6) Splitting
> 7) Elbowing
> 8) Shouldering
> 9) Advancing
> 10) Withdrawing
> 11) Looking-Left

12) Gazing-Right

13) Central-Equilibrium.

In brief, the Eight Postures are the basis for all Taijiquan postures. The Five Activities are the functions applied within each of postures. Hence, there are not really Thirteen Postures. It would probably be better to translate this as "The Thirteen Principle Functions."

"This type of solo posture practice was performed from ancient times up to Yang Jianhou in the final years of the Qing dynasty (清代, 1644–1912). It was handed down from teacher to pupil. Its importance should be quite evident."

Cai Tui Exercise

"Within the boxing arts is the Pulling Leg (採腿, Cai Tui) method and the much more vicious Flying Leg (翅腿, Chi Tui) method. Flying Leg uses the toes and a high climbing kick to your opponent. Cai Tui employs the sole of the foot to strike the opponent's knee cap or to go directly into the shin bone. It is used in a similar manner to picking up the foot to walk. The power of this method is great and all who experience its ferocity suffer serious injury."

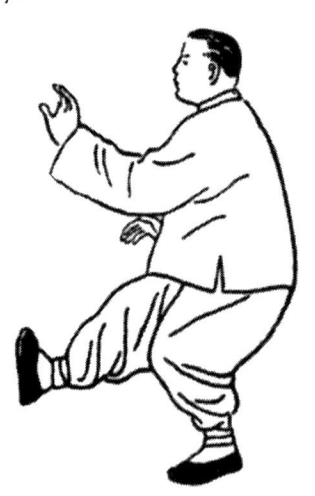

The meaning of *Cai* is to pluck, like with a flower, where one hand holds the base of the stem and the other hand plucks the flower. *Tui* means "leg." This exercise is the basis for the Taijiquan postures that employ a kick. This method is a combination of Expressing the Qi and Post exercises.

Flying Leg is a method developed by the Shaolin martial art school. The kick in this method is directed to the opponent's head, whereas in Cai Tui the attack method is directed to affect the opponent's knee, arm, and head simultaneously.

"There are many applications of this kicking technique within Taijiquan, yet few really understand the true function. Fearful of injury when engaging with an opponent, so at best they seek only types of kicks that are considered safe and solid. But without training the Cai Tui method, they really cannot accomplish even those types of kicks.

"The training method is to first use the right foot [standing on the left leg] and employ a pulling motion to an opponent with the right hand, which does the work of leading and grasping the wrist [of the opponent's incoming punch toward the rear], pulling his arm forward and downward diagonally. The left palm is used to strike forward, like lightning toward the opponent's face, yet keeping the hand and arm in a slightly bent position. Simultaneously, the sole of the right foot is moved as if being pulled forward and down [onto the opponent's knee cap or shin bone]. When pulling, the body is turned slightly sideways and moved down into a slight squatting position. Both hands are simultaneously opened toward the front and back. The left knee is slightly bent and the weight is entirely on the left leg.

"In the upper body, the chest is hollowed and the back raised, the Qi is sunk into the Dan-Tian, a light and sensitive energy is retained on top of the head, and the waist is seated and the pelvic area relaxed.

"When it is the left foot that performs Cai Tui, the left hand does the work of leading and grasping. The right palm is extended to the opponent's face like lightning. The left foot is simultaneously moved forward and down to perform Cai. The right knee is bent slightly and the weight is placed entirely upon it. The remainder is like that in the previous right-leg style.

"These types, the left and right styles of Cai Tui, should be practiced together [don't just practice one side]. After a long period of training the entire body will undergo a change and the four limbs will be able to move as one unit externally. Also, the waist and legs will acquire Seated Energy (坐勁, Zuo Jin). Otherwise, when wanting to kick an opponent, one foot will not rise properly because the other foot will be floating. Thus, the opponent will not be knocked down, but you yourself will have fallen over.

"Train in these solo styles of Cai Tui, for if you learn them you will not be caught unawares."

> The technique involved in the exercise holds true for all kicks trained and employed in Taijiquan practice. The main principle being that when kicking with one leg, the other leg sinks so it doesn't follow the upward movement and float up. Otherwise, balance is lost and it will be easy for an opponent to grab the kicking leg and so knock you over.
>
> Another distinctly Taijiquan principle is being expressed here—to ensure the opponent is defeated, all three levels of his body are being affected. First, the *upper portion* of his body is being startled with a strike to his face, causing him to rise and lean back. Second, the *middle portion* of his body, the arm, is being pulled forward and downward diagonally, causing him to lean forward and his waist moved into a defective position. Third, the *lower portion* of his body, his forward leg and knee, is pushed back causing him to fall back. The idea of affecting these three portions of the body

simultaneously—upper, middle, and lower—is seen in every technique of Taijiquan practical application, as it ensures the opponent cannot maintain a sense of balance and is always led to a defective position.

It is interesting that Bruce Lee himself had incorporated the use of Cai Tui. Even though in his movies he performed high kicks, he reportedly thought that in a real situation a kick should never be performed higher than the waist because it allowed an opponent to seize the leg too easily. Many martial artists, Bruce Lee included, would practice this Cai Tui in a unique manner. Tying a rope around one ankle, with the rope looped through a pulley high on a wall, they would use the arms to pull the rope back and down diagonally, thus causing the leg to kick upward without any muscular force. Meaning, they trained themselves to kick naturally and spontaneously when the arms used a Pulling technique.

What is more important is that the text says, "the entire body will undergo a change." The change implied here is that by continued practice of Cai Tui the legs will acquire intrinsic energy (Seated Energy) and the Qi can then be expressed in the legs as well. So whether or not you are interested in the martial aspect of this technique, it is still a very important Qigong method and should not be passed over.

Chapter Six
Meditation

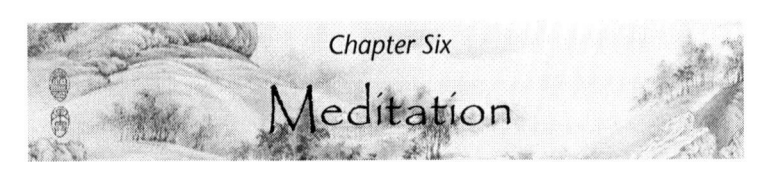

靜 坐

The instructions within this chapter are unique, as the methods for visualizing Qi points, or cavities, are very old, coming from a Ming Dynasty sect of Daoism. In present-day Qigong terminology, the Lesser Heavenly Circuit (sometimes called "Microcosmic Orbit") is what this text refers to, in older terminology, as Before Heaven Qi and After Heaven Qi, which are located in the Upper Dan-Tian (head and neck area), Middle Dan-Tian (between the chest and navel), and the Lower Dan-Tian (navel and lower abdominal area). These methods are very effective for stimulating Qi, and should be approached in stages.

"People should be aware that meditation can be very beneficial. On a minor level it can nourish the body [for health]; on a greater level you can enter the gate of a skilled cultivator [for attaining longevity and immortality].

"It is certain that with proper meditation practice many significant attainments will ensue; consequently, you must actively seek to acquire stillness internally. However, by no means is this stillness similar to the idea of motionlessness."

Stillness is ultimately a state of mind, whether one is performing the movements of Taijiquan or seated in meditation. Stillness is internal, whereas motionlessness is external. Stillness of the mind means that the mind (rational thinking) is emptied, while the Mind-Intent is then functional—meaning, there is heightened perception, inner awareness, and so on.

"The meditational aspect of Taijiquan is to seek stillness within movement. Mentally, they both have the same flavor; consequently, Taijiquan practice has the same attainments as meditation. Both of these actively seek internal stillness. The two are identical paths.

"Moreover, the rise and descent of the breath within Taijiquan practice creates a complete orbit of the Before Heaven Qi, which is identical to the secret of the *Golden Elixir* (金丹, Jin Dan) within meditation practice. Within Daoist alchemy this Golden Elixir is also called the *Pill of Immortality* (仙丸, Xian Wan), which is produced by disciplining and refining the Three Treasures [Jing, Qi, and Shen]. This is also the very essence and goal of Taijiquan to produce this Golden Elixir.

"It is said of those who cultivate the Dao through just seated meditation: 'Sitting for long periods, there is a fear that the pulses [Qi flow] will accidentally become obstructed because seated meditation can cause an excess of Qi in the meridians.' But by means of the Taijiquan exercises the internal Qi is assisted in its circulation. This is most certainly not an empty or false statement. An old, often stated Daoist verse says, 'To cultivate the Dao without first cultivating the body is useless.'

"Internal cultivation [of the Three Treasures] is called 'the foremost stage of cultivation.' Within this process are three levels of cultivation: great accomplishment, middle accomplishment, and minor accomplishment. Even though there are these three divisions of accomplishment, in the end they are the same."

> Great accomplishment is the full achievement of the "Immortal Spirit"—to be an immortal. Middle accomplishment is forming and congealing the "Golden Elixir" (Jing, Qi, and Shen). The minor accomplishment is experiencing "Free Circulation of Qi" and "Accumulating Qi in the Dan-Tian."
>
> These are said to be the same because they are a progression of accomplishment, starting with the minor accomplishment.

Civil and Martial Cultivation

"Civil cultivation is internal and martial cultivation is external. The internal physical culture is the disciplining of the Jing, Qi, and Shen. Martial matters (practicing the boxing arts) are the external culture. But through cultivating both of these you can completely unite the internal and external aspects, the inside and outside, figuratively. To do so is a high level of achievement.

"The lowest level is to just have knowledge of the civil, its physical culture and attainments, or to know just the martial matters and attainments, on a solely intellectual basis.

"Meditation and civil cultivation are one; therefore, meditation and Taiji share a very close relationship. An ancient ode says, 'Contemplate without disturbance.' Another saying is, 'Stillness is benevolence.' Meng Zi said, 'Just do not move the mind.' All of these verses on stillness are extremely important. When you can sit in stillness, the mind will become level and the Qi will circulate harmoniously. The Mind-Intent will cause the body to remain upright, and all your thoughts will be clear and tranquil. Then at the time when engaged in Sensing-Hands, it will not matter what intrinsic energy is employed as it will not be coming from a confused mind."

Kung Fu Zi (公夫子, Confucius, 551–479 B.C.) is one of China's greatest sages and most influential philosophers whose teachings formed Confucianism, one of China's three great teachings along with Daoism and Buddhism. His famous statements "Meditate without disturbance" (思無邪, Si Wu Xie) and "Stillness is benevolence" (仁者靜, Ren Zhe Jing) reveal that only through internal stillness and tranquility can one truly be kind, compassionate, and humane, because a still mind has no greed or selfishness.

Mencius (孟子, Meng Zi, born 372 B.C.) was an ardent supporter of Confucianism. His work, *The Book of Mencius,* forms the fourth book in the Confucian Classics. His statement, "Just do not move the mind," (不動心, Bu Dong Xin) literally means, "Do not make use of the rational thinking mind."

"The method for stilling the mind consists primarily of controlling your temper. Control means to harness your courage, which is internal [not arrogance, which is external]. With robust courage the Qi will be strengthened. If the courage is not robust, then the spirit [Shen] will be weak.

"So at the time of performing the meditation exercises you can become very confused. Not only might you not progress but you may harm yourself. If possible, you should follow the orthodox practice [the teachings handed down from founder to master, to student, and so on]. Following this is just as important concerning Taiji practice. This will prevent the spreading of corrupt practices."

Seated Meditation Qigong

"The correct manner for sitting is the full lotus [both legs crossed and placed on opposite thighs], half lotus [one leg crossed with the foot placed on the opposite thigh], or the common seated posture [with legs crossed but not placed on the thighs]. Any of these will do."

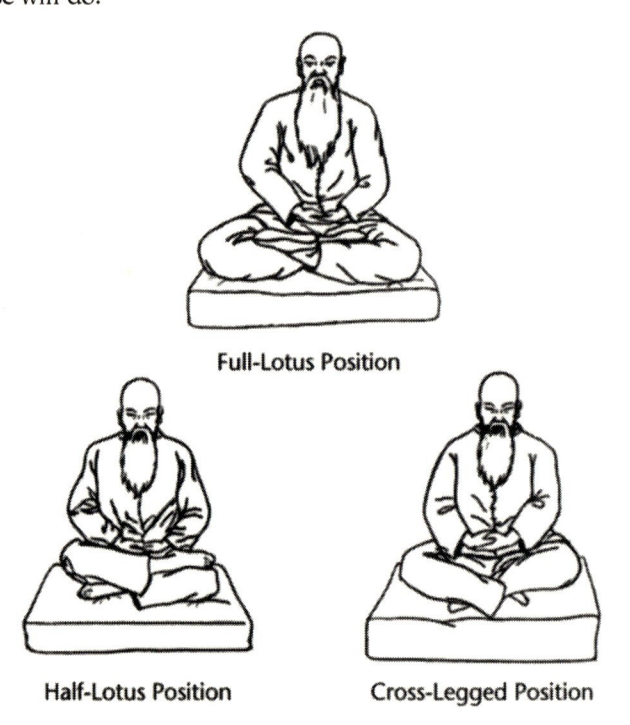

Full-Lotus Position

Half-Lotus Position

Cross-Legged Position

See *"Qigong Teachings of a Taoist Immortal"* by Stuart Alve Olson for further explanation of seated meditation postures.

"It is necessary to suspend the head to keep the body upright [retain a light and sensitive energy on top of the head], sink the shoulders and hollow the chest. Relax and open the entire body. Place the tongue up against the roof of the mouth. The lips and teeth press lightly together. Slightly close both eyes. This is called, 'letting down the screens.' Regarding the two hands—place the back of the left palm in the center of the right palm close to the front of the lower abdomen [Dan-Tian], lightly and loosely above the thighs."

"Afterward, when the mind and thoughts are settled and the navel region is relaxed, when there is no 'I' or 'others,' and all confused thinking is utterly ignored, then you can bring an end to the constant examining and turn back the hearing [employ internal listening, rather than external hearing]. In a common Daoist saying it is stated, 'Be ever cautious to put a stop to the Five Thieves.'"

> The last paragraph points out the benefits of stillness in relation to the Five Activities (五行, Wu-Xing: Metal, Fire, Wood, Water, and Earth), which permeate Daoist philosophy (and all Chinese thought). Wu-Xing has been somewhat erroneously translated as "Five Elements;" however, the underlying idea here is not so much the material substance of elements, rather the activities of the elements.
>
> The *Five Thieves* negatively affect the *Five Viscera*. But through stillness and internal cultivation, these Five Viscera can be positively affected by the Five Spiritual Energies. The following chart will elucidate this further.

Five Thieves	Five Viscera	Five Spiritual Energies
Joy	Heart	Shen (Spirit)
Anger	Liver	Hun (Heavenly Spirit)
Pleasure	Lungs	Po (Earthly Spirit)
Grief	Spleen* (or abdomen)	Yi (Mind-Intent• and Qi)
Lust	Kidneys	Jing (Regenerative)

- The spleen and Mind-Intent are identical to the abdomen and Qi respectively. It is a matter of discretion as to the terminology.

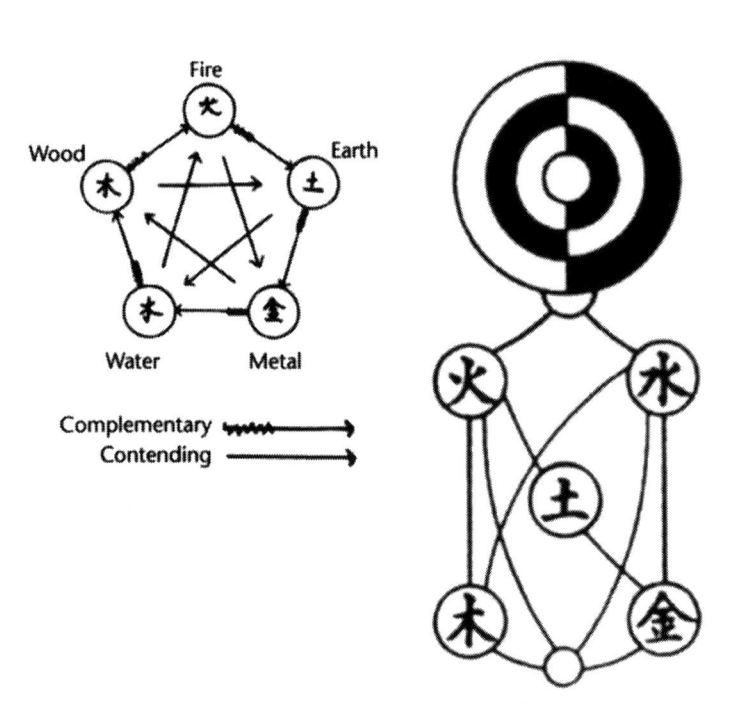

"Pay heed to the ears and the result will be ears that do not listen externally; then the sexual energy (精, Jing) can be restored in the kidneys (腎, Shen).

"Pay heed to the eyes and the result will be eyes that do not gaze externally; then the spirit (魂, Hun, Heavenly Spirit) can be restored in the liver (肝, Gan)."

"Pay heed to the mouth and the result will be tacit understanding without speech; then the spirit (神, Shen) can be restored in the heart (心, Xin).

"Pay heed to the nose and the result will be a nose that does not smell externally; then the spirit (魄, Po, Earthly Spirit) can be restored in the lungs (肺, Fei).

"Pay heed to the mind and then, when the 'Mind-Intent' is applied, it will be Limitless (無極, Wu Ji); then the Mind-Intent (意, Yi) can be restored to the spleen (脾, Pi).

"Jing (regenerative energy), Shen (human spirit), Hun (Heavenly spirit), Po (Earthly spirit), Yi (Mind-Intent), Xin (heart), Gan (liver), Fei (lungs), Pi (spleen), and Shen (kidneys) —each will undergo restoration; each will return to their natural state. This results in a natural manifestation of the Heavenly Mind (天心, Tian Xin), where yet another state of perception arises."

Tian Xin, literally "a Heavenly Mind," a boundless and limitless state of mind.

"The time periods for meditation should be once in the morning after waking and once before bedtime. If you have spare time in the afternoon, you should meditate once then also. It does not matter whether the periods are long or short; for

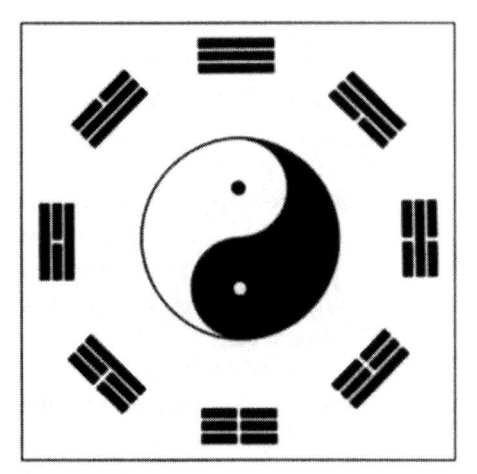

Taiji double fish symbol in conjunction with the Eight Diagram arrangement created by Fu Xi.

example, one quarter of an hour, one half hour or even one full hour—any of these will suffice.

"With sitting you can attain delightful states. The entire body, internally and externally, will be exceptionally comfortable and pleasing. Within the mouth, the tongue is depressed [up against the palate]. This will cause the saliva to gush forth, which will taste sweet and pleasant when swallowed. This is called 'the completion of fire and water,' the unification of the mercury and lead [the elixir] or Qian (乾, Heaven, ☰) and Kun (坤, Earth, ☷)."

Unlike Western notions of saliva being a negative substance, Daoists and Buddhists view it as a valuable substance for health and spiritual cultivation, calling it "Amrita," "Jade Juice," "Sweet Nectar," and "Divine Water." The Qi (fire, or heat, in the lower abdomen) uniting with the saliva (water), which is gulped down into the Dan-Tian (the cauldron). In

Daoist alchemy, ingesting saliva and breath are two important practices.

Qian *(The Creative,* Heavenly principle) Kun *(The Receptive,* Earthly principle) are terms from the *Yi Jing* (易經, *Book of Changes).* Qian, ☰, represents Yang in its highest aspect; Kun, ☷, represents Yin in its highest aspect.

"When beginning to learn seated meditation, the four limbs will become agitated and uncomfortable. Thoughts will be wild and it will be difficult to stop the thinking process. Even after a long time they will stop and then go; but naturally, over a course of time, you will be able to get rid of them.

"When beginning to learn, it is absolutely necessary to pay attention to one's inability to activate the Qi. Breathe only through the nose. Seek to master this naturally. To activate the Qi it is necessary to achieve this through proper regulation of the breath. Then, and only then, can you train the Qi. Otherwise, it will be easy to form a corrupt practice in which the Mind-Intent causes the Qi to rise upward, resulting in congestion in the brain. Eventually, you will suffer from a disorder in the nervous system. The spirit will be divided internally, causing suffering from heart and stomach ailments. If the spirit should fall, then you may suffer from bleeding piles, irregular bowel movements, or a ruptured hernia.

"The benefits of seated meditation follow after a long period of practice. When everything unites at the aperture and navel, then the Qi can be circulated. This is great accomplishment kung fu, but you cannot accomplish it without the true orthodox teaching."

Four Methods of Circulating Qi

"The following are the proper methods for mobilizing and circulating the Qi."

With each Qi cavity, visualize it as a very bright, pulsing, and white ball or disc, expanding to about a 3-inch diameter on the inhalation, and shrinking to half size when exhaling. Qi meridians should be visualized as something on the size of a garden hose and as whitish in color. When inhaling, visualize the Qi flowing through half the circuit (as indicated in the diagrams), and then exhale visualizing the last half of the circuit. So as not to confuse the reader, when visualizing the Qi in the meridians you don't need to bother visualizing the cavities, just have a mental image of leading the Qi through the area of the cavity. Conversely, when just visualizing the Qi cavities there is no need to visualize the Qi meridians that connect them. In analogy, visualizing Qi cavities is like focusing on a kink in a garden hose, so that the obstruction can be eliminated. Visualizing on Qi meridians is like focusing on the water flowing freely through the garden hose.

Another aspect of these training methods is that the circuits should be done both in clockwise and counterclockwise manners. The instructions herein are for the clockwise motion of visualizing Qi cavities and Qi meridians, but they should also be reversed. So even though the instructions might say, "perform nine complete circuits," you will actually do eighteen complete circuits.

Keep in mind that the intent of all these methods is not so much a specialized technique, rather they are for getting the meditator to exercise their visualization skills. Much like someone who physically exercises to develop better muscle tone, many drills are used, not just one. So it is with developing Qi.

When first seating yourself and right before practicing any of the methods you should initially perform nine Cleansing Breaths. Train yourself progressively, taking the time and patience for results to be experienced. Do not just intermix the methods and jump from one to another. Only practice one of the methods per session, and at first use only Natural Breathing. During each session, first complete nine circuits (eighteen when counting both directions) focusing on the cavities, then practice visualizing Qi coursing through the meridians for nine (eighteen) circuits. When you acquire some sense of heat in the abdomen, then move on to the practice of Reverse Breathing until you experience heat in the middle of the back. After this use Natural Breathing with Heng Ha (inaudibly so the sounds are heard internally only) until you can sense heat on top of the head and begin seeing flashes of light in the mind's eye. It is at this point that you will then want to begin practicing Holding the Breath on each Qi cavity, breathing in and out on each cavity (breathe in and hold the breath in the first cavity of the first circuit, for three or nine heartbeats, then exhale. Then inhale again, hold the breath on the next cavity, and continue in this manner through all the cavities of each circuit until the Qi can be felt moving like water through a hose.

Practice each of the four methods in this manner, first using Natural Breathing with each circuit until achieving some accomplishment. For example, even if it takes six

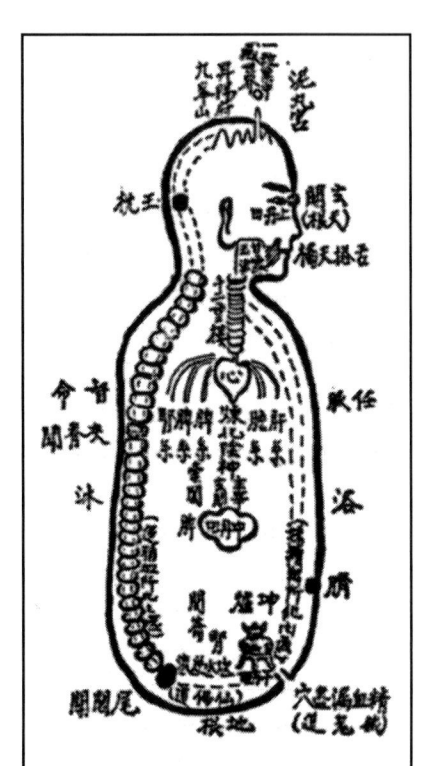

Original diagram of the Xian Tian and Hou Tian circuit, according to the Daoist sect Long Men (Dragon Door).

months or more just doing the Natural Breathing before experiencing results, then do so. Only after experiencing results should you move on to the next breathing method. Each period of sitting should be no shorter than twenty-minutes, but an hour is best, and you should do so at least twice a day. For each sitting session use only one type of breathing method—do not be interchanging them during the sitting time. When the effects of Natural Breathing are easily sensed—then and only then—move on to the next type of breathing method.

By practicing in this way, you will eventually enter the stage of the "One Breath," where the Qi and breath will be completely mobilized by the Mind-Intent.

Method One: Circuit for After Heaven Breathing

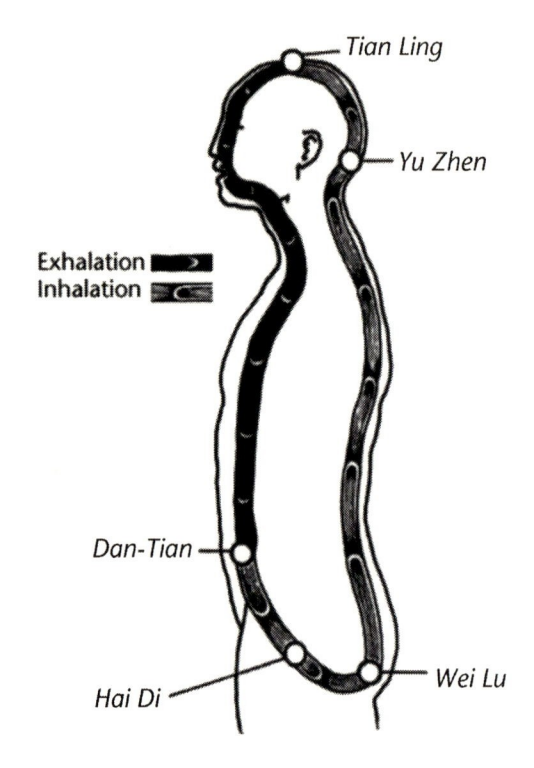

Tian Ling
Yu Zhen
Exhalation
Inhalation
Dan-Tian
Hai Di
Wei Lu

"Within Taiji, the After Heaven Circuit of Qi is distinct from the Before Heaven Circuit of Qi. They are, however, also alike; it is just the direction and path of circulation of Qi that is different."

[Inhale]
"From the Dan-Tian, the Qi passes down through the Sea Bottom (海底, Hai Di—coccyx area) directly over to the Tail Gate (尾閭, Wei Lu), and then upward along the spine. It then

passes through the Jade Pillow (玉枕, Yu Zhen), and flows along the top of the head to the Spirit of Heaven (天靈, Tian Ling)."

[Exhale]
"Moving downward along the front of the forehead to the raphe of the upper lip, it flows through the [Adam's apple] into the pit of the stomach, and then into the navel, thus returning to the Dan-Tian."

> With this method, just continue to breathe and pay as close attention as possible to each cavity mentioned, so the breath is kept low in the abdomen. Some might wonder how to focus on a Qi cavity or meridian while simultaneously paying attention to the breath in the lower abdomen? This is really quite simple in function. At the beginning of sitting and preparing to visualize the Qi, just put your Mind-Intention into the lower abdomen. The breath will stay there, but if you sense the breath has risen up to the solar plexus region or into the lungs, then just stop the visualization and return the breath to the lower abdomen again. Too many meditators are not taught to constantly be correcting themselves while sitting. Whether it be the breath or posture, always stop the method at hand to correct these two aspects. Zen master Dogen equated correcting the posture and breathing as being the primary cause of achieving enlightenment.

Method Two: Circuit for Before Heaven Breathing

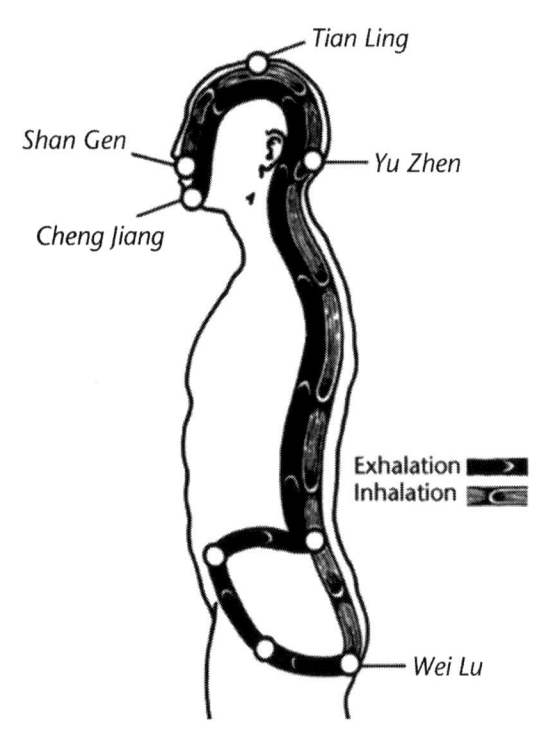

[Inhale]
"From the Base of the Mountain (山根, Shan Gen) the Qi moves upward to the Spirit of Heaven (Tian Ling). Pressing on in reverse motion, the Qi moves down, passing through the Jade Pillow (Yu Zhen), and down along the spine until reaching the Tail Gate (Wei Lu).

[Exhale]
The Qi then rises up through the intestinal region into the Dan-Tian, then, moving directly across, it returns to connect with the

back of the spine and moves upward. Passing through the Jade Pillow and Spirit of Heaven it again moves down along the front of the head through the Base of the Mountain and then into the Fluid Container (承漿, Cheng Jiang) cavity. Swallow the saliva. The Qi then returns to the Dan-Tian."

> In this method the saliva is stirred in the mouth by the tongue nine times after the completion of nine circuits. Stirring the saliva is simply a matter of rotating the tongue nine times (clockwise) inside the mouth over the gums, then sucking the collected saliva back and forth nine times along the tongue. The saliva is then swallowed like a hard object being gulped down into the lower abdomen. When doing so stretch the neck upward slightly to make sure its passage is clear.

Method Three: Lesser Heavenly Circuits (小周天, Xiao Zhou Tian)

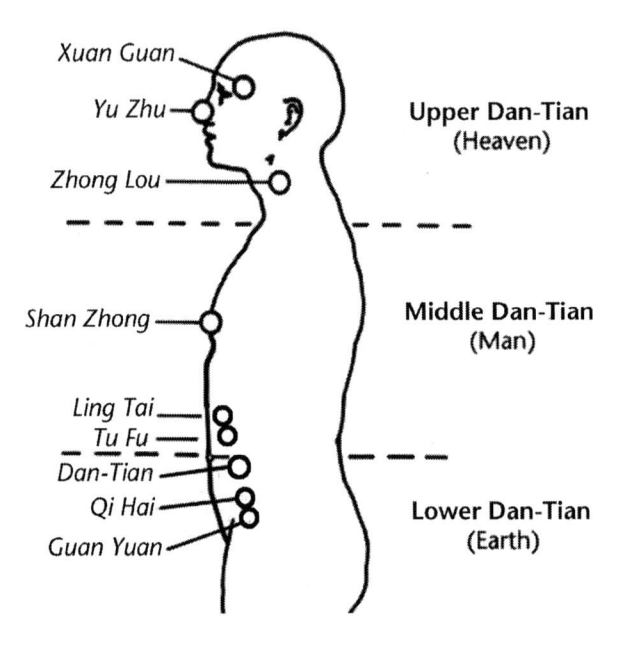

```
Xuan Guan
Yu Zhu                    Upper Dan-Tian
                              (Heaven)
Zhong Lou

Shan Zhong                Middle Dan-Tian
                              (Man)

Ling Tai
Tu Fu
Dan-Tian
Qi Hai                    Lower Dan-Tian
Guan Yuan                     (Earth)
```

"Upper Dan-Tian Circuit (上丹天周, Shang Dan Tian Zhou)

"1) Begin this circuit in the Upper Dan-Tian, or Mysterious Pass (玄關, Xuan Guan) cavity, between the two eyes and slightly upward about 3 centimeters.

"2) Then move to the Jade Pillar (玉柱 Yu Zhu) cavity, at the tip of the nose.

"3) Lastly, move to the Big Tower (重樓, Zhong Lou) cavity, by the great protrusion [Adam's apple] and hollow [area beneath it]."

Repeat the process by moving your attention back to the Mysterious Pass. Doing so until nine circuits have been completed.

"Middle Dan-Tian Circuit (中丹天周, Zhong Dan Tian Zhou)

1) Begin this circuit in the Middle Dan-Tian, or Inner Deer (膻中, Shan Zhong) cavity, between the bones which resemble the character for man, 人 (Jen).

2) Then move to the Spiritual Terrace (靈台, Ling Tai) cavity, at the navel and up 1.5 inches.

3) Earthen Cauldron (土釜, Tu Fu) cavity, 8 centimeters up from the navel."

> Repeat the process by moving your attention back to the Inner Deer. Doing so until nine circuits have been completed.

"Lower Dan-Tian Circuit (下丹田周, Xia Dan Tian Zhou)

1) Begin this circuit in the Lower Dan-Tian (Field of Elixir) cavity [3 inches behind the navel].

2) Then move to the Ocean of Qi (氣海, Qi Hai) cavity [2 inches below the Field of Elixir].

3) Lastly, move to the Original Pass (關元, Guan Yuan) cavity [3 inches below the Field of Elixir].'"

> Repeat the process by moving your attention back to the Field of Elixir. Doing so until nine circuits have been completed.

"Each of these three openings in each circuit should be visualized as having a 3-inch diameter."

> The visualization of Upper, Middle, and Lower Circuits, (called the Lesser Heavenly Circuits) are three separated practices, and are not really circuits as such. They are just individual visualizations on each of the three Qi cavities in each circuit. They are to be performed successively from

Upper, Middle, to Lower Dan-Tian areas. All that is required of this method is to first visualize the breath pulsing in the Qi cavity as described, doing so nine times, and then moving on to the next Qi cavity. So for one circuit, there will be twenty-seven breaths, and each circuit is repeated nine times.

Do all three circuits successively, starting with the Upper Dan-Tian Circuit, then the Middle Dan-Tian Circuit, and ending with the Lower Dan-Tian Circuit.

Method Four: Greater Heavenly Circuit (大周天, Da Zhou Tian)

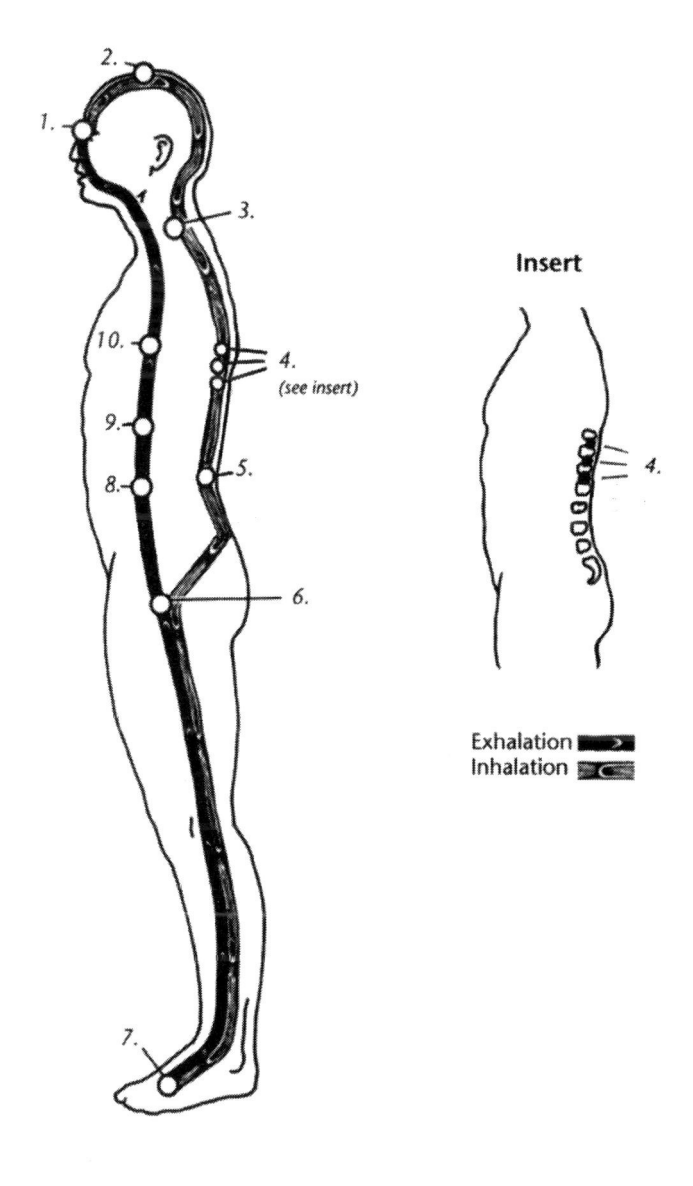

Insert

Exhalation
Inhalation

[Inhale]

"1. From the Illimitable (無極, Wu Ji) to the Hall Seal (印堂, Yin Tang, the space between the two eyebrows) and the Supreme Ultimate (太極, Taiji, at the angle of the sun and moon, the two eyes)."

> This is all directed at focusing on the "Mysterious Pass," in more common Daoist terminology an area at the very top of the bridge of the nose between the two eyes.

"2. *Embrace the Sun and Moon* (at a direct angle from the sun and moon) upward to the Kunlun (崑崙, the topmost point on top of the center of the head)."

> Normally called the Mud Pellet (泥丸, Ni-Wan) cavity.

"3. *Ride a Black Ox Through the Dark Valley Pass* (in the neck, behind the two, soft, fleshy areas—the center of the two sides of this point)."

> In the neck behind the top bone joint of the neck.

"4. *Directly Arrive at Heaven's Heart* [the spaces between the three protruding joints in the middle of the back]."

> This area is the same as the Double Pass (雙關, Shuang Guan) cavity, directly in the middle of the back.

"5. *Small Rest at the Center of Mt. Xu Mi* (須彌山, Xu Mi Shan, on both sides of the waist)."

> The two hollow areas where the kidneys reside.

"6. *Seeing a Dragon at the Bottom of the Sea* (yin in front, yin behind—the soft, fleshy space between)."

The perineum, between the anal opening and base of the genitals.

[Exhale]

"7. *Inner Field* (在田, Zai Tian, to both Bubbling-Well [湧泉, Yong Quan] points by moving downward on the back of the legs)."

On the bottoms of both feet, back about 1 inch from the balls of the feet and in the center of the foot.

At this point the exhale finishes in the Bubbling-Well cavities, and the inhalation then starts its ascent of Qi from this point as well.

"8. *Plant the Jade, Rest, and Plow* (behind the navel, 7 centimeters; in front of the spine 3 centimeters. Return through the back of the legs, stopping to rest with an inhalation and exhalation)."

The lower Dan-Tian region.

"9. *Ten-Thousand Images* (萬象, Wan Xiang, between the two openings)."

The middle Dan-Tian region or middle stomach area.

"10. *Returning to Spring* (囘春, Hui Chun, below the *Big Tower* [and] above the *Inner Deer*, within the upper front of the middle of the chest—solar plexus region)."

Then continue the exhale directly into the Wu Ji cavity again. After nine such circulations, stir the saliva nine times, swallow, and begin nine more circuits again.

Even though the diagram shows the man standing, the circuit is completed in a seated posture. It would be too difficult to show the placement of the Qi cavities and meridians if showing a seated figure. It is important to note that the halfway point of this circuit is in the feet, not the Dan-Tian or top of the head. This particular practice is sometimes referred to in Daoism as "breathing through the heels." It is very important to your progress to train this method of visualizing the Qi cavities and Qi circulation through the indicated Qi meridians. Many Daoists and martial artists have failed in their discipline on this method, with the result that in old age their legs grow weak from lack of Qi circulation.

Concluding Comments

"The Qi within men's bodies is like a fiery sphere, and so lead the Qi to follow the reverse revolutions of circuits as well. Ultimately, both circuits are natural. Concerning seated meditation and fixed concentration, the motive is enlightenment; good roots will appear and culminate in great achievement. In every man exists this nature [of enlightenment and good roots]. Therefore, in the practice of Taiji and in seeking to attain the skills inherent to it, compose a plan to cultivate the mind and body simultaneously; otherwise, the training of seated meditation and kung fu will accomplish little.

"It is essential to know that the Dao of sitting takes many years, as it does with learning and practicing Taiji. Seated exercises act as an aid, but it is insufficient in itself for acquiring the intrinsic energy skills of Taiji.

"How much training does it take to accomplish all this? If you take the door of shortcuts there will be no progress. It is as if trying to measure nine mountains, but *'To fail in completion by one basketful.'* [to fall short of a goal]. How unfortunate!"

About Stuart Alve Olson

Stuart Alve Olson is the head teacher and cofounder of the Sanctuary of Dao, where he focuses on translating various Daoist texts, conducting lectures, leading retreats, and teaching.

Stuart began studying Asian culture and language in the late 1960s, but started no formal training until 1979 when he went to Gold Mountain Monastery in San Francisco.

In 1979, he formally took Triple Refuge with Chan Master Hsuan Hua, receiving his disciple name Upasaka Kuo Ao.

In 1981, he began participating in the meditation sessions and sutra lectures given by Dainin Katagiri Roshi at the Minnesota Center for Zen Meditation.

In the spring of 1982, Stuart undertook a Buddhist bowing pilgrimage, "Nine Steps One Bow," from the Minnesota Zen Center to the border of Nebraska, ending the practice after two and a half years. During this time, he began living full-time with Master T.T. Liang, studying Taijiquan, Daoism, Praying Mantis Kung Fu, and Chinese language under his tutelage.

In 1992, Stuart furthered his studies of Praying Mantis Kung Fu with Master Kong Wei (恭衛功夫師) in Indonesia.

Presently, Stuart lives and teaches in Phoenix, Arizona, where he is helping operate the Sanctuary of Dao and Valley Spirit Arts, the publishing company for his works. You can email him at contact@valleyspiritarts.com.

His body of works include:

Chen Kung Series
Tai Ji Jin: The Intrinsic Energies of Taijiquan, Valley Spirit Arts, 2013
Tai Chi Sword, Saber, and Staff, Valley Spirit Arts, 2011
T'ai Chi Sensing-Hands—A Complete Guide to T'ai Chi T'ui Shou Training from Original Yang Family Records (Available soon from Valley Spirit Arts, 2013)

Other Taijiquan Books
Tai Ji Quan Treatise, Valley Spirit Arts, 2011
Steal My Art—The Life and Times of Tai Chi Master T.T. Liang, North Atlantic Books, 2002
T'ai Chi According to the I Ching—Embodying the Principles of the Book of Changes, Healing Arts Press, 2002
T'ai Chi for Kids: Move with the Animals, Illustrated by Gregory Crawford, Bear Cub Books, 2001
Imagination Becomes Reality: 150-Posture Taijiquan of Master T. T. Liang, Valley Spirit Arts, 2011
The Wind Sweeps Away the Plum Blossoms: Yang Style Taijiquan Staff and Spear Techniques, Valley Spirit Arts, 2011
T'ai Chi Thirteen Sword: A Sword Master's Manual, Unique Publications, 1999

Daoist Books
The Jade Emperor's Mind Seal Classic: The Taoist Guide to Health, Longevity, and Immortality, Inner Traditions, 2003

Tao of No Stress: Three Simple Paths, Healing Arts Press, 2002
Qigong Teachings of a Taoist Immortal: The Eight Essential Exercises of Master Li Ching-Yun, Healing Arts Press, 2002

Kung-Fu Books
The Complete Guide to Northern Praying Mantis Kung Fu, Blue Snake Books, 2005, 2010

Suggested Reading

T'ai Chi Ch'uan: For Health and Self-Defense Philosophy and Practice by Master T.T. Liang. Vintage Press, 1977.

Fundamentals of T'ai Chi Ch'uan by WenShan Huang. South Sky Book Co., 1973.

The Tao of Tai Chi Chuan: Way to Rejuvenation by Jou, Tsung Hwa. Charles E. Tuttle, Co., 1981

T'ai Chi Ch'uan and Meditation by Da Liu. Schocken Books, 1986

Cheng Tzu's Thirteen Treatises on T'ai Chi Ch'uan by Cheng Man Ch'ing. Translated by Benjamin Pang Jeng Lo and Martin Inn. North Atlantic Books, 1985.

T'ai Chi: The "Supreme Ultimate" Exercise for Health, Sport and Self-Defense by Cheng Manch'ing and Robert W. Smith. Charles E. Tuttle, Co., 1967

T'aichi Touchstones: Yang Family Secret Transmissions. Compiled and Translated by Douglas Wile. Sweet Ch'i Press, 1983.

T'ai Chi Ch'uan: The Technique of Power by Tem Horwitz and Susan Kimmelman with H.H. Lui. Chicago Review Press, 1976.

Practical Use of T'ai Chi Ch'uan (Its Applications and Variations) by Yeung (Yang) Sau Chung. T'ai Chi Co., 1976.

Lee's Modified T'ai Chi for Health by Lee Yingarng. Unicorn Press, 1958.

Yang Style Taijiquan. Editor: Yu Shenquan. Hai Feng Publishing Co., 1988.

Wu Style Taijiquan by Wang Peisheng and Zeng Weiqi. Hai Feng Publishing Co., 1983.

Chen Style Taijiquan. Compiled by Zhaohua Publishing House. Hai Feng Publishing Co., 1984.

About the Sanctuary of Dao

The Sanctuary of Dao is an educational, spiritual, and literary organization dedicated to the preservation and propagation of Daoism. Materials on Daoism are produced and distributed, along with in-depth commentaries to help people apply Daoist teachings to their lives and practices. Offering services to its members and the public in the form of Dao Talks, Daoist texts and lectures, meditation sessions, and retreats, the Sanctuary of Dao also provides teachings through a number of courses on a range of Daoist subjects.

All these various teachings are offered so as to create skilled and knowledgeable students of Daoist self-cultivation. It is not a matter of cultivating just one aspect of the self, but the entire self. It is no small matter when Lao Zi states, "It is because of the transformation of a person that it is called 'obtaining the Dao.'"

Please visit our website at sanctuaryofdao.org for more information about our organization and programs.